Dr. Susan's Solutions: Healthy Menopause

Womens Wellness Publishing, LLC
www.womenswellnesspublishing.com
www.facebook.com/wwpublishing

Mention of specific companies or products in this book does not suggest endorsement by the author or publisher. Internet addresses and telephone numbers for resources provided in this book were accurate at the time it went to press.

Cover design by Rebecca Rose

ISBN 978-1-939013-86-6

Note: The information in this book is meant to complement the advice and guidance of your physician, not replace it. It is very important that women who have medical problems be evaluated by a physician. If you are under the care of a physician, you should discuss any major changes in your regimen with him or her. Because this is a book and not a medical consultation, keep in mind that the information presented here may not apply in your particular case. In view of individual medical requirements, new research, and government regulations, it is the responsibility of the reader to validate health practices and treatments with a physician or health service.

D1208769

Acknowledgements

I want to give a huge thanks to my amazing editors Kendra Chun and Sandra K. Friend for their incredibly helpful assistance with putting this book together. I also greatly appreciate my fantastic Creative Director, Rebecca Richards, as well as Letitia Truslow, my wonderful Director of Media Relations. I enjoyed working with all of them and found their help indispensable in creating this exceptional book for women.

Table of Contents

Introduction

Dear Friend,

I know that you are reading this book because you are looking for positive and effective solutions for menopause. I have written this book just for you, to share with you the all natural treatment program that I have developed and successfully treated thousands of my patients.

I have been working with menopause related issues with my patients since I first started my clinical practice. As a physician specializing in alternative and complementary medicine, I have heard numerous questions from concerned women about how best to deal with their own particular set of symptoms. This decision has no "one right answer."

How Women Differ in Their Need for Menopause Relief

Each woman dealing with menopause symptoms in my medical practice has had her own unique set of issues. I have found that some women with severe symptoms such as hot flashes, night sweats, vaginal dryness or mood swings are looking for instant relief. Other women with escalating risk factors, due to their hormonal changes, are more concerned about how to prevent longer-term health problems, such as osteoporosis and heart disease, for which they are at risk.

Many of my own patients, however, have been very concerned about using conventional hormone replacement therapy (HRT) to relieve their menopause symptoms. They have been worried that HRT could intensify serious preexisting health problems such as uterine cancer, heavy bleeding from uterine fibroid tumors, severe migraine headaches, or blood clotting problems.

Other women, free of illness, have feared that the long term use of synthetic and animal derived hormones may accelerate the onset of a disease for which they are at risk, based on a strong family history. This concern occurs most often among women whose mothers or sisters have had breast cancer or heart disease. Some of my patients have tried HRT but experienced unacceptable side effects such as depression, breast tenderness, or fluid retention that occur no matter how the estrogen was given or at what dosage. As a result, they were completely turned-off by HRT and didn't want to use it again.

Many research studies done over the past ten to fifteen have confirmed the negative effects that HRT can have on a woman's health. As these studies have continued to accumulate, the use of alternative therapies have become more and more appealing to the millions of women who are trying the find relief from their menopause symptoms that is both safe and effective.

Approximately fifteen to twenty percent of menopausal women in developed countries like the United States have no menopause symptoms or their symptoms are so mild that they manage well without HRT. Some women refuse to use HRT on a philosophical basis, even if they could benefit from it, preferring instead to pursue nondrug treatment options such as nutritional therapies and acupuncture.

What Millions of Women Are Facing Today

The dilemma that my own patients have dealt with regarding menopause therapy mirrors the struggles of many other women in our country. Most often, a woman with menopausal symptoms goes to her physician and hears that she may either choose hormonal replacement therapy (HRT) or not. Yet, millions of women today are also concerned about using HRT and, like my patients, have rejected this option. In fact, the number of women between the ages of 45 to 54 grew more than 50 percent between 1990 and 2010. It is currently estimated that 50 million women in the United States are in menopause – women who are currently struggling with this issue.

An article published in *Family Practice News*, states that there has never been a time in the U.S. when more than 35 percent of menopausal women have opted to use hormone replacement therapy. Recent studies support these findings stating that HRT use is as low as 8 percent in some parts of the country. The most common reasons for women to stop hormone therapy are menstrual-like bleeding, the fear that the increased hormones will increase their risk of developing breast cancer, weight gain and bloating, or ineffectiveness of the therapy to adequately control their symptoms. Another study of more than 2000 women found that the majority had either ceased using the hormones entirely or had significantly cut their originally prescribed dosage.

With 80 to 85 percent of all menopausal women symptomatic to some degree, most women could benefit from some type of treatment, either prescription hormones or alternative therapies. Many women simply do not know enough about the other treatment options available to them, or they are uncertain about the right path to choose.

The Purpose of This Book

I have written this book to share with you information about the wonderful alternative therapies and bioidentical hormone regimens that have greatly helped many thousands of my own patients be free from uncomfortable and, even disabling, symptoms of menopause. I have seen so many women regain their sense of well-being and joy of living, free from symptoms that I wanted to share my programs with you.

In this book, I share with you the many alternative therapy treatment options that I have found can produce effective menopause relief. Menopause doesn't just affect our physical body but also our emotional well-being, our ability to deal with stress and even our mental clarity. Often, I have found with my own patients that one single therapy option may not be enough to restore a woman to the level of physical, emotional, and mental comfort and well-being that she desires to enjoy her life to the fullest.

Luckily, a woman need not choose one option to the exclusion of all others. In my own clinical practice, many patients have benefited from my programs in which they combined supportive and helpful nutritional supplement programs, healthful dietary changes, improved exercise habits, as well as learning how to handle day-to-day stress better. Some of my patients have also benefited greatly from the use of bioidentical hormones.

Often, they have become far healthier using this combined approach than they could ever be following only one treatment option. Not only were their hormones healthier but also their entire health status was greatly improved on all levels, physical, mental and emotional.

To help you develop the best treatment program for yourself, I have included in this book much of the information I have shared over the years with women who have seen me as patients or attended my classes. I have included many therapies and techniques that have benefited my own patients who have given me much helpful and positive feedback. It is also based on the best medical research in this field and contains the most exciting, up-to-date information on the newest all-natural therapies.

In reading through this book, I recommend that you use the therapies that appeal to you and interest you the most. You will probably enjoy working with them and receive the most benefit. I have included chapters on diet, natural plant sources of estrogen, vitamins, minerals, essential fatty acids and herbs. There are also sections on acupressure, stretches, physical exercise and stress reduction techniques as well as bioidentical hormones.

I hope that you enjoy working with the information and programs in this book as much as I have enjoyed sharing them with you.

To a joyful and healthy life!

Love,

Dr. Susan

Part I:
Female Hormones and the Symptoms of Menopause

1

How Female Hormones Function

Our body produces three hormones that support the normal functioning of the reproductive tract and menstrual cycle. These powerful hormones help regulate not only body chemistry but also physical characteristics such as skin texture, muscle tone and body shape. The two female hormones that we make in substantial amounts during our active childbearing years are estrogen and progesterone. We also make very small amounts of male hormones, androgens, which affect our female functions. An example of such a hormone is testosterone. In this chapter, I discuss these hormones and their role in female development.

If you don't want to read about the science of hormones and their production, you can skip this chapter and go on to the next chapter to learn about the menopause health evaluation.

What Are Hormones?

Hormones are chemicals secreted by glands in the body. Once a hormone is released into the bloodstream, it may circulate to a target gland. The hormone acts as a messenger, instructing the target gland to make its own hormone. In some instances, a hormone triggers chemical reactions in different parts of the body. The body makes dozens of hormones, most of which are outside the scope of this book, because they regulate functions unrelated to the reproductive system.

For example, some hormones regulate how efficiently we can fight off viral and bacterial infections, while others regulate digestive processes. Still other hormones help our bodies manage stressful situations effectively by regulating muscle tension and blood flow to vital organs.

In this book, I'll be focusing on the three major hormones that we produce as women, estrogen, progesterone and testosterone since they play a vital role in maintaining our health and well-being throughout life. When the production of these sex hormones diminishes greatly with menopause, we are significantly affected, physically, mentally and emotionally.

How Estrogen Affects the Body

As mentioned earlier, estrogen enters the cells of many different tissues and stimulates chemical reactions and physiological changes. Let us look at how estrogen affects our sexual organs and the physical characteristics that we tend to think of as specifically female.

First of all, estrogen causes the growth of our sexual organs. During childhood, we produce estrogen in only small amounts. During puberty, estrogen production increases twentyfold or more. With the increased estrogenic stimulation, female sexual organs begin to change into those of adult women. Our uterus, vagina and fallopian tubes increase in size; our external genitals enlarge. Our vaginal and urinary tract linings thicken and become much more resistant to trauma and infection. This is important in adulthood when women become sexually active. With estrogen stimulation, the lining of the uterus thickens and the endometrial glands develop—necessary to nourish a fertilized egg during the early stages of pregnancy.

In addition to causing maturation of the female sexual organs, estrogen causes an increase in overall body fat. This is particularly pronounced in the buttocks, hips and breasts, contributing to the softly rounded female contours that we associate with sexual maturation. Estrogen is responsible for the disposition of fat under the skin, giving rise to the soft and fine-textured skin that many women enjoy during their younger years. Estrogen also causes fluid and salt retention in the tissues, which additionally helps to plump up and fill out our skin.

Estrogen has an important effect on promoting bone health. It helps retain calcium in the bones thereby protecting against bone loss. By reducing the levels of low-density lipoprotein (LDL) in the body and elevating the levels of the protective blood fats, estrogen protects women from developing heart attacks and strokes. These "good" fats are called the high-density lipoproteins (HDL). Also, estrogen has a direct positive effect on the endothelial lining of the blood vessels, as well as affecting dozens of other physiological functions as varied as blood sugar level, emotional balance and memory.

How Progesterone Affects the Body

As mentioned earlier, progesterone is primarily produced by the corpus luteum (yellow body) of the ovary. It is also secreted in high doses by the placenta if a pregnancy occurs. Though estrogen primarily causes tissues to grow and thicken, progesterone has a maturing and growth-limiting effect on the tissues of the body. For example, progesterone prevents the uterine lining from thickening to the point where menstrual bleeding becomes too profuse and long lasting.

Progesterone also stimulates secretory activity in the body. For example, under the stimulation of progesterone during the second half of the menstrual cycle, the uterine lining secretes nutrients needed by the developing embryo if pregnancy occurs. Progesterone also triggers the production of secretions in the fallopian tube. These secretions are important for the nutrition of the fertilized egg as it moves through the fallopian tube prior to implantation in the uterus. In breast tissue, progesterone causes certain cells to become secretory in their function, which is necessary if the breasts are eventually to produce milk for nursing an infant.

The production of progesterone at mid-cycle causes an increase in body temperature by about one-half to one degree Fahrenheit. Many women monitor this temperature change to assess their fertility during the time of expected ovulation. Like estrogen, progesterone has an effect on many physical and chemical functions in the body.

These effects often oppose and complement those of estrogen. For example, progesterone acts as a sedative on the nervous system. When progesterone levels are too high, it can cause depression and fatigue. In contrast, estrogen has a stimulatory effect on the nervous system. High levels of estrogen can trigger anxiety, irritability, and mood swings.

Progesterone tends to elevate the blood sugar level, while estrogen lowers it. Thus, the healthy balance between the two female hormones is very important.

How Androgens Affect the Body

As mentioned earlier, women secrete small amounts of androgens or male hormones. Both the ovaries and adrenal glands secrete small amounts of testosterone. Both of these glands manufacture testosterone from a precursor hormone called androstenedione. Like estrogen and progesterone, the level of androstenedione varies throughout the menstrual cycle. The level rises at mid-cycle, when androstenedione is secreted from the ovarian follicle, and during the second half of the menstrual cycle when it is produced by the corpus luteum (which also secretes progesterone).

The secretion of small amounts of androgens is very important for female health. They help in maintaining our sex drive. Women who are placed on the oral estrogen/testosterone combination for HRT or testosterone cream for various health problems may note a significant increase in their sexual drive. Androgens also help maintain muscle strength as well as vaginal lubrication and elasticity. In fact, testosterone cream is sometimes applied directly to the vaginal tissues as a treatment for vaginal atrophy. It must be used carefully, however, because side effects of excessive androgen use can include masculinization such as deepening of the voice or growth of excessive facial hair.

How DHEA Affects the Body

While ninety percent of this hormone is produced by the adrenal glands, a small amount is produced by the ovaries as a precursor to the production of estrogen, progesterone, and androgens. Cholesterol is the basic building material for the production of all male and female hormones. Through a series of biochemical steps, cholesterol is converted first to a precursor hormone called pregnenolone. The pregnenolone is then converted, via either of two pathways, to DHEA or progesterone. These pathways then merge to form testosterone and, finally, estrogen. Thus DHEA acts as a precursor hormone in the ovarian production of male and female hormones. DHEA, whether from adrenal or ovarian sources, is present in higher concentrations than any other hormone in the body. It is also converted into adrenal stress hormones.

Blood levels of DHEA peak when a woman is in her twenties and decreases in a linear fashion thereafter. Like estrogen, progesterone, and androgens, the decrease in DHEA accelerates after menopause. By age seventy, DHEA levels are barely detectable.

Low levels of DHEA have been linked to accelerated aging, a higher risk of breast cancer, and cardiovascular disease. Recent studies have found DHEA to be beneficial in cases of obesity, memory loss, bone density, hot flashes, and cardiovascular function. DHEA is available by prescription. Until very recently it was thought that wild yam was converted into DHEA in the body. But research has shown that this is not true. Current studies show that Pro-Gest cream, a topical progesterone, does increase DHEA levels.

Hormone Production During the Menstrual Cycle

Certain glands such as the ovaries, adrenals, pituitary, and hypothalamus assume a major role in producing and regulating levels of the three hormones estrogen, progesterone, and androgens. These hormones regulate the menstrual cycle and later in life, determine how easily we make the transition through menopause. Other glands, such as the thyroid, also play a supporting role. Let us look at how they produce our female hormones, first during our active reproductive years and then how this process changes as we approach menopause.

I begin by discussing the normal menstrual cycle and how it functions. This information will help you understand the normal ebb and flow of our female hormones throughout the month. Once we reach menopause, this cycle changes as the production of our hormones diminish greatly.

First, let's understand why menstruation occurs. Menstruation refers to the shedding of the uterine lining, or endometrium. Each month the uterus prepares a thick, blood-rich cushion to nourish and house a fertilized egg. If conception occurs, the embryo implants itself in the uterine lining after six or seven days. If pregnancy does not occur, the egg does not implant in the uterus and the extra buildup of uterine lining is not needed. The uterus cleanses itself by releasing the extra blood and tissue so the buildup can recur the following month.

The mechanism that regulates the buildup and shedding of the uterine lining is controlled by fluctuations in hormonal levels. These fluctuations are based on a feedback system. When the ovaries secrete high levels of estrogen and progesterone, this "turns off" production of hypothalamic and pituitary hormones that normally stimulate ovarian function. Conversely, when ovarian production of estrogen and progesterone are low, the hypothalamic and pituitary hormone production rises in an attempt to stimulate the ovaries to work harder.

How does the feedback system operate in the menstrual cycle? The initial trigger for the menstrual cycle comes from hormones produced in the hypothalamus, a walnut-sized collection of highly specialized brain cells located above the pituitary. The hypothalamus regulates many basic bodily functions in addition to the production of female sex hormones, including temperature control, sleep patterns, thirst and hunger. The hypothalamus is very sensitive to stress such as emotional problems and infections. Severe stress can affect the ability of the hypothalamus to pass signals to the pituitary and on to the other endocrine glands. This can cause an imbalance in the menstrual cycle.

The pituitary, located at the base of the brain, stimulates all the glands of the body and provides the next mechanism that regulates the menstrual cycle. To communicate with the pituitary, the hypothalamus releases messengers into the bloodstream called FSH-RF (follicle-stimulating hormone-releasing factor) and LH-RF (luteinizing hormone-releasing factor). When these messages from the hypothalamus are received, the pituitary begins to produce its own hormones, which trigger the menstrual cycle and ovulation by secreting FSH (follicle-stimulating hormone) and LH (luteinizing hormone). The pituitary also triggers adrenal function through the production of ACTH (adrenocorticotropic hormone) and thyroid function through TSH (thyroid-stimulating hormone).

Once FSH and LH are released into the bloodstream, their destinations are the ovaries, the female reproductive organ. The ovaries are two small, almond-shaped glands located in a woman's pelvis. The ovaries hold all the eggs a woman will ever have, in an inactive form called follicles. At birth, each female may have as many as 1 million follicles. By puberty, the number of eggs has been reduced to 300,000 to 400,000. The eggs decrease in number throughout a woman's life, until menopause, at which time the follicles have atrophied and lost their ability to produce estrogen. Without sufficient estrogen, menstruation ceases.

Each month, FSH and LH from the pituitary cause the follicles to ripen and the release of an egg for possible fertilization. (Usually, only one ovary is stimulated in a cycle.) In doing so, the follicles begin to produce the hormones estrogen and progesterone. Estrogen reaches its peak during the first half of the cycle, while progesterone output occurs after mid-cycle when ovulation has occurred.

Following menstruation, during the first half of the menstrual cycle, the endometrium, or uterine lining, gradually rebuilds itself. Estrogen causes the glands of the endometrium to begin to grow long; the lining thickens through an increase in the number of blood vessels, as well as the production of a mesh of fibers that interconnect throughout the lining. By mid-cycle, the lining of the uterus has increased three times in thickness and has a greatly increased blood supply.

After mid-cycle, usually around day 14 in a 28 day cycle, ovulation occurs. Ovulation refers to the production of a mature egg cell, which is capable of being fertilized. Normally, the mature egg finds its way to a fallopian tube for the journey to the uterus. The follicle that produced the egg for that month (or Graafian follicle) is further stimulated after mid-cycle by LH and changes into the yellow body, or corpus luteum. The corpus luteum secretes progesterone—the second ovarian hormone of the menstrual cycle. Progesterone helps prepare the uterine lining for a possible pregnancy. With stimulation by progesterone, the uterine lining secretes glycogen (a storage form of sugar), mucous, and other substances needed to sustain a fertilized egg. Progesterone also causes a coiling of the blood vessels and the uterine lining becomes swollen and tortuous.

If the egg is fertilized, it will implant on the uterine wall and the corpus luteum will continue to secrete progesterone. If no fertilization occurs, the corpus luteum begins to deteriorate and the progesterone and estrogen levels decrease. The lining of the uterus starts to break down and menstruation begins. With the onset of menstruation, the monthly ebb and flow of hormones begins again.

Hormone Balance in the Body

When the levels of estrogen and progesterone are optimally balanced throughout the month, female menstrual and reproductive health is the result. However, optimal function not only depends on how much of each hormone is produced, but also on how efficiently the body metabolizes and disposes of the hormones. Once they have done their job, they no longer need to remain in the body.

Normally, the hormones are metabolized and broken down by the liver. This occurs as they pass through the liver while circulating in the bloodstream. For example, when liver function is healthy and efficient it will transform the main type of estrogen secreted by the ovary, called estradiol, into other forms of estrogen. Estradiol is a chemically active and efficient form of estrogen. It binds to many tissues such as the uterus, breasts, and ovaries, as well as the brain, heart and other organ systems in the body through specific estrogen receptors that allow it to enter into the cells. As a potent form of estrogen, estradiol stimulates many chemical reactions in the target tissues.

However, as with everything in life, proper balance is important. When estradiol is present in too high an amount or for too prolonged a period of time, it can cause adverse reactions in the body. Research studies suggest that, when unopposed, it may be carcinogenic to estrogen-sensitive tissues such as the breast and uterus.

The liver prevents excessive build-up of estradiol in the blood circulation by inactivating it. The liver converts estradiol to a less active, intermediary form called estrone and finally to estriol, a very weak form of estrogen. Like estradiol, these weaker forms of estrogen can also bind to estrogen receptors in the cells. However, their physiological effects on the body are less pronounced.

Although estrone is also a carcinogenic form of estrogen, medical research studies suggest that estriol may actually decrease our susceptibility toward developing female-related cancers such as breast cancer. Estradiol is 12 times more potent than estrone and 80 times more potent than estriol. Thus, the total estrogenic effect of estradiol is many times greater than the other two forms combined; therefore, smaller doses are needed.

When the liver is healthy, the conversion process occurs quite efficiently. However, poor nutritional habits can compromise healthy liver function. The intake of too much alcohol, fat, or sugar can impair the liver's ability to handle the overload of food as well as the breakdown of the female hormones. In addition, research studies have shown that a lack of sufficient B vitamins adversely affects estrogen metabolism.

Estrogen passes from the liver via the bile into the intestinal tract. Again, diet affects how estrogen is handled in the intestinal tract. When a woman eats a high-fat, low-fiber diet, the dietary fat stimulates the growth of certain types of bacteria in the intestinal tract. These bacteria chemically change the breakdown products of estrogen into forms that can be reabsorbed back into the body. As with poor liver function, this process elevates the levels of estrone and estradiol in the bloodstream.

In contrast, a low-fat, high-fiber diet promotes excretion of estrogen by the body. High dietary fiber binds with estrogen in the intestinal tract and helps remove it from the body in bowel movements. Estrogen is also excreted from the body through the urinary tract.

Hormone Production During Menopause

As women reach their early forties, the reproductive tract begins to show signs of aging. By this time, most women have ovulated regularly for almost 30 years. With each ovulation, one follicle matures for a possible pregnancy. However, an additional 1000 follicles or more degenerate with each menstrual cycle and lose their ability to be fertilized. At this rate, most women have exhausted their supply of follicles by their late forties or early fifties.

As the number of follicles diminishes, the remaining follicles produce less estrogen. During the cycles when the follicles don't mature to ovulation, progesterone production is insufficient or absent. In fact, during the transition to menopause, ovulation occurs with decreasing frequency. Because of this drop in hormonal output by the ovaries, the pituitary hormone FSH rises in an attempt to drive the ovary to secrete more estrogen.

Sometimes the high levels of FSH can overstimulate the remaining follicles to produce an abundance of estrogen. In such cycles, a woman may produce very high levels of estrogen yet not produce progesterone because the follicles never mature sufficiently. The tendency for estrogen to fluctuate between low and high levels of production can continue throughout the menopause transition and may last from one to seven years.

During this time, women are very vulnerable to developing a variety of health problems. The imbalance in the estrogen and progesterone levels can trigger the growth of uterine fibroids, PMS symptoms, and changes in the amount and frequency of the menstrual cycle. Women whose estrogen level drops tend to have longer intervals between periods, with lighter bleeding, before stopping entirely.

Women who have temporary surges in estrogen levels prior to menopause without the secretion of progesterone may have increasingly heavy and more frequent menstrual bleeding. The menstrual cycle often becomes irregular. This can be a very difficult time for some women and they are faced with the need for close monitoring by their physician when symptoms are severe. These symptoms present problems such as bleeding or fibroid growth, which may lead to more hysterectomies in this age group.

Finally, as the follicles become exhausted, the estrogen drops to a level at which there is not enough of this hormone to build up the lining of the uterus sufficiently to induce menstruation. A woman is officially considered to be menopausal when she has had no menstrual period for at least six months. For most women, this occurs between the ages of 46 to 53. Some women, however, may experience menopause as early as their thirties or as late as age 59; the average age is 52.

As estrogen levels diminish, the level of FSH begins to rise, finally attaining levels considered to be diagnostic for menopause. FSH continues to remain high during the postmenopausal years. In fact, physicians often monitor FSH levels to determine the onset of menopause.

During the postmenopausal years, the body does continue to produce small amounts of estrogen. Even though the follicles are exhausted, another part of the ovary called the stroma can still make small amounts of estrogen. The stroma is the supportive tissue of the ovary that helps provide structure to the gland. In addition, the body can also make estrogen by converting the male precursor hormone, androstenedione, to estrogen.

Though androstenedione is made by the adrenal glands, its conversion to estrogen occurs in the body's fat cells. Obese women make more estrogen after menopause because they have more fat cells. In fact, some women may make enough estrogen to delay aging of the skin, vagina, bladder, breasts, and other tissue for a decade or so. Thinner women tend to show loss of estrogen support earlier, as do women with less active adrenal or ovarian stromal output of hormones. By the time women reach their seventies and eighties, however, even these small extra sources of estrogen begin to diminish. As the hormonal support falls to lower and lower levels, the female body gradually ages during the years following menopause.

In the early postmenopausal years, common symptoms of diminished hormonal output include hot flashes, night sweats, vaginal and bladder atrophy, mood swings and fatigue. The lack of hormonal support can increase the risk of osteoporosis, heart attacks, adverse lipid and vessel wall changes, and stroke.

These symptoms and health issues will be discussed in depth in the following chapters in terms of the treatment and prevention benefits that bioidentical hormone replacement therapy (HRT) and alternative therapies can provide.

2

The Menopause Health Evaluation

Once you have entered menopause, I recommend that you schedule an initial health evaluation with your physician to identify any undiagnosed health issues that can then be adequately treated. A health evaluation may vary in its components depending on your medical status and what specific menopause related health problems your physician is most concerned about. Tests used in evaluating a woman in menopause may include the following:

- A complete physical examination, including a pelvic exam and a breast exam. A PAP smear to determine a cancerous or precancerous lesion of the cervix.

- Blood tests to check liver function, blood sugar, cholesterol, triglyceride, calcium, and phosphorus levels, as well as tests of thyroid function. Complete blood count to check for anemia, as well as a urinalysis.

- Mammography and professional breast examination to check for breast cancer. Mammograms done by experienced radiologists are capable of detecting 90 percent of all breast cancers.

- Bone density studies (dual x-ray absorptiometry, DEXA) to help determine the level of bone loss. This is an important test for women who may be at higher risk for osteoporosis.

- A review of your family medical history to gather clues about your risk of cardiovascular disease, osteoporosis, and breast and other cancers.

- If you have vaginal bleeding after menopause, an endometrial biopsy or vaginal ultrasound may be done to check for hyperplasia (overgrowth) of the uterine lining and endometrial cancer. A progesterone challenge test may also be done after menopause to check for endometrial hyperplasia.

Most physicians recommend annual visits. At this time, you should discuss any symptoms that you may have. Your blood pressure will normally be monitored at each visit and a breast and pelvic exam done to check the health of these tissues. Most importantly, it is an excellent time to ask your doctor any questions that you may be concerned about therapies for your symptoms.

If you are not satisfied with your physician's answers or feel that your physician is standoffish or abrupt, you may wish to seek another opinion or doctor in your community. Unexpressed concerns that are not discussed with your physician may delay the diagnosis and treatment of health problems that can arise during the course of treatment. The best results occur when a true partnership exists between doctor and patient.

Testing your Hormone Levels

The method for checking women's hormone levels had severe limitations until the 1990's. A single blood sample was taken and analyzed, though the results of this one-time check were less than optimal. In addition, the stress of having blood drawn was enough to throw off a woman's hormone levels and skew the results.

Fortunately, there are saliva female hormone tests that are non-invasive (no needle sticks!) and highly accurate. These tests can take the guesswork out of making a proper diagnosis and make it possible to design individualized treatment that delivers maximum benefit with minimum risk of side effects.

Best of all, saliva hormone testing is accessible. Even physicians who still don't routinely order saliva hormone testing will usually write an order when a patient requests it. You can even order a limited saliva hormone test kit on your own directly from a laboratory, without a doctor's order.

Saliva Versus Blood

Like blood, saliva closely mirrors hormone levels in your body's tissues. However, saliva is a particularly accurate indicator of free (unbound) hormone levels. This is the key, as only free hormones are active, meaning that they can affect the hormone-sensitive tissues in your breasts, brain, heart, and uterus. Saliva testing therefore provides a superior measure of the levels of hormones that actually affect vital body systems, mood, tissue levels of sodium and fluid, and many other important functions.

Additionally, blood testing only provides a one-time "snapshot" of hormone levels, whereas saliva testing provides a dynamic picture of hormonal ebb and flow over an entire menstrual cycle. In fact, 11 samples are collected during the month, all at the same time of day, and then sent to a laboratory. The lab measures and charts your progesterone and estradiol (your most prevalent and potent form of estrogen) levels. These results are then compared to normal patterns.

Finally, saliva testing is easy, stress-free and non-invasive. You can collect your own saliva samples, which means you don't have to go to your doctor's office or a lab. Plus, there's no need to draw blood.

Get Tested

If you think saliva hormone testing is right for you, consider consulting your physician. Having your doctor order the test has two advantages: The profile is more extensive, and your insurance may cover the cost. Several laboratories perform the test; in the event your physician does not have a preference, I recommend Genova Diagnostics (gdx.net or 800-522-4762), as well as ZRT Laboratory (zrtlab.com or 866-600-1636). If your doctor doesn't order the test, or you simply want insight to help you develop your own self-care regimen, you can order a test kit from several sources. Aeron Laboratories has a wonderful Life Cycles saliva test kit (aeron.com or 800-631-7900).

When you get your test results, you'll want to pay particular attention to your estradiol levels. A reading of one to two pico grams per milliliter (pg/ml) indicates that you are menopausal.

3

Hot Flashes

Hot flashes and other vasomotor symptoms are the most common complaints surrounding menopause. These symptoms refer to brief episodes of heat and perspiration that usually begin to occur as the menstrual periods cease. In fact, 80 percent of American women experience hot flashes, with 40 percent of these women having symptoms severe enough to seek medical care. This high prevalence of hot flashes is seen in menopausal women throughout the Western world including Canada and Europe.

Variations in Hot Flash Incidence

Interestingly enough, the pattern we see in the Western world is not duplicated in many other cultures. Far fewer Japanese and Indonesian women experience hot flashes, with an incidence of only 10 to 15 percent. Mayan women living in the Yucatan in Mexico do not experience hot flashes at all. Their only symptom as they move into menopause appears to be menstrual cycle irregularities. A number of interesting studies suggest that this difference in prevalence of hot flashes is probably due to dietary factors. Women in Asian, Mayan, African and other cultures consume much higher levels of estrogen-containing plant-based foods than women in Western societies. Thus, even though their own levels of estrogen diminish at menopause, women in these other societies receive significant hormonal support from their diet.

Women in our country who do not suffer from hot flashes tend to eat a more vegetarian-based diet high in plant estrogens. Also, women who carry excess body weight may have fewer problems with hot flashes. This is because women with a greater mass of fat cells can continue to produce a form of estrogen called estrone. Estrone is manufactured from a precursor hormone called androstenedione made by the adrenal glands. This additional source of estrogen can be significant enough to prevent hot flashes in heavier women, even after their main source of estrogen, estradiol, has diminished in output from the ovaries. Conversely, thin women who carry less body fat may suffer more intensely from hot flashes.

Although most women don't begin to have hot flashes until they have ceased menstruating, 15 to 20 percent of women suffer from hot flashes during transition when they are still having a menstrual cycle. In addition, women who have gone through an abrupt, surgical menopause with removal of ovaries and uterus have a higher incidence of hot flashes than do women who undergo natural menopause. If not started on HRT, women who have had surgical menopause can suffer from severe, frequent hot flashes.

Symptoms of Hot Flashes

Many women sense a hot flash beginning a few seconds before it starts. Most women describe the hot flash itself as a sudden and intense episode of warmth and heat. These episodes arrive unexpectedly, and the woman suddenly notices that she feels very warm. The hot flashes usually begin above the waist, especially on the chest, face and neck, and then radiate to other parts of the body. The blood vessels of the skin dilate when the hot flash is occurring, causing the skin to become pink and rosy colored.

The hot flashes are often accompanied by varying amounts of sweating— mild in some women and profuse in others. With more severe episodes, women may become so wet that they have to change their clothes or bed sheets. After the initial period of warmth, the sweat cools down the skin temperature, causing shivering. This temperature instability may be very uncomfortable for many women, causing them to alternately shed or add clothes.

The temperature changes that women feel have been evaluated in research studies. These studies have found measurable changes in skin temperature just before the hot flash begins. In addition, there is a 10 to 15 percent increase in pulse rate.

The hot flash usually lasts from 30 seconds to 5 minutes. However, in extreme cases, patients report hot flashes lasting as long as an hour.

Frequency also varies. Some notice them infrequently, having only a few a year or once or twice a month. Many women will have hot flashes on a daily basis. Three and four episodes a day are not unusual, with 30 to 40 hot flashes a day occurring in severe cases. Other women may have several hot flashes during the night.

When hot flashes recur throughout the night, sleep is often disturbed. Many women wake up from a sound sleep feeling hot and perspiring profusely. Often it is difficult to go back to sleep. Women with menopause-related insomnia may feel exhausted during the day because of sleep deprivation. Insomnia is a very common reason for women to visit their doctors seeking relief.

Other Vasomotor Symptoms

Women who have hot flashes often have other symptoms as well. Like hot flashes, these symptoms are due to vasomotor instability (varying degrees of vasoconstriction and vasodilatation of the blood vessels) and thus are considered to arise from the same cause. Such symptoms may present odd sensations that can be quite worrisome to women who do not understand that they are menopause related; for most women, they diminish in time.

These symptoms include nausea, dizziness, faintness and palpitations (rapid and forceful heartbeats). Some women notice strange sensations of numbness and tingling in their arms and fingers. An unusual symptom is formication, which women describe as a crawling feeling all over their skin. Luckily, this is not a common symptom.

Luckily, hot flashes do not last forever for most women. For half of the menopausal women who experience these symptoms, hot flash symptoms disappear within a year. For another 30 percent of women, they last up to two and one-half years. Unfortunately, however, for 20 percent of women, the hot flashes and other vasomotor symptoms can last five to ten years or even longer.

Cause of Hot Flashes

The cause of hot flashes is unclear, but it may be related to the decrease in estrogen output at the time of menopause. The pituitary gland responds to the drop in estrogen and progesterone by increasing its level of gonadotropins, FSH and LH, in an effort to elevate estrogen and progesterone levels. The pituitary, in turn, is stimulated by releasing factors from the hypothalamus, which also regulates temperature control. As a result, the hormonal instability occurring at this time may also cause the "thermostat" in the brain to be reset downward with menopause. Another hypothesis is that hot flashes occur when the estrogen receptors in the hypothalamus do not receive enough estrogenic stimulation. In response, they may release a chemical substance that produces the hot flashes and other vasomotor responses.

Whatever the mechanism, lack of estrogen appears to play a major part in producing hot flashes, through its role in nervous system function and its effect on blood vessels. Research studies show that estrogen both excites and inhibits warm and cold sensitive nerve cells in the hypothalamus. Estrogen and progesterone are known to affect body temperature during the menstrual cycle. In blood vessels, estrogen can moderate vascular tone and affect how blood flow is distributed to various parts of the body. Women with hot flashes have higher blood flow to their forearm than women without hot flashes. Once they are treated with estrogen, the forearm blood flow diminishes.

Hot Flash Triggers

Although the main cause of hot flashes appears to be the hormonal and nervous system instability that occurs at the time of menopause, other factors such as environment, emotions and diet can also trigger hot flashes. Women often report that the intensity and frequency of hot flashes increase in warm weather. During the worst heat of the summer, women may stand in front of air conditioners or open refrigerators to find relief. Often they wear as few layer of clothing as possible. Many women keep a thermos of ice-cold water or other beverages close by to cool themselves down.

Stress often brings on hot flashes. Patients report that the incidence of hot flashes increases dramatically before a talk or formal presentation, before a trip, during times of job or family stress, or even with strenuous exercise. In addition, the use of alcohol or caffeinated foods and beverages such as coffee, black tea, cola drinks and chocolate can trigger hot flashes because they tend to dilate the blood vessels. Spicy food or hot drinks may have the same effect.

Women who suffer from frequent and intense hot flashes should endeavor to keep a calm and peaceful mindset and practice meditation or relaxation techniques. They should also pay close attention to their diet during this period. Many self-help techniques to relieve hot flashes are discussed in the alternative therapy section of this book.

Attention to diet, specific nutritional supplements and practicing stress reduction techniques have all been found to be very effective for the relief of hot flashes and are described later on in this book.

4

Vaginal & Bladder Aging

The reduced estrogen and androgen output by the ovaries after menopause causes the vagina and bladder to age dramatically, compromising their ability to function normally. Unlike hot flashes, mood swings and other early symptoms of menopause that tend to diminish over time, the symptoms of vaginal and bladder aging increase. As the years pass, they can cause women severe discomfort.

After a discussion of these changes and the symptoms that can result, information will be presented later on in this book about the many helpful therapies that relieve these symptoms. Some therapies even reverse the signs of tissue aging and return the vagina and bladder to more youthful and healthful states.

Vaginal and Bladder Changes After Menopause

With the onset of menopause, estrogen levels can drop by as much as 75 percent. As mentioned earlier, estrogen causes dilatation and relaxation of the blood vessels, promoting good blood circulation to the organs and tissues throughout the body. When estrogen levels dwindle, blood flow to the genitals decreases. The tissues lose their pink or rosy color and, over time, become paler. The vagina has many estrogen receptors, so its tissues are very responsive to the levels of hormones available. When estrogen is deficient, the vaginal and urethral linings lose their thick protective layer of surface cells and become thinner, drier and less elastic. They are much more easily injured and traumatized.

One of the earliest signs of vaginal aging is loss of lubrication. The cervix and vagina secrete much less mucus. How soon this occurs depends on how much estrogen the body makes after menopause. Within five years of menopause, 25 percent of women suffer from vaginal dryness because their ovaries and adrenals lose the ability to make sufficient estrogen to support these tissues. In other women whose bodies continue to make small but helpful amounts of estrogen, it may take as long as ten years before vaginal dryness becomes a problem. But eventually, it occurs in all women. An active sex life does help to maintain vaginal health and keep dryness to a minimum for a longer time.

Although vaginal and urethral dryness and a tendency toward being easily traumatized and irritated are early signs of vaginal and bladder aging, these are by no means the only indications. With time, the vagina actually shrinks and becomes shorter and narrower at the opening. The vaginal walls become less elastic. Patients have told me that they approach sex cautiously because their vaginal opening is so narrowed that penetration is quite painful.

Symptoms of Vaginal and Bladder Aging

As you can imagine, these changes in the vagina and bladder cause uncomfortable symptoms that affect normal function. These symptoms include vaginal soreness and painful intercourse, loss of sexual desire, vaginal and bladder infections and stress incontinence.

Vaginal Soreness and Painful Intercourse

With the thinning and narrowing of the vagina, penetration can be a painful experience. Many women find that their annual pelvic examination and PAP smear become quite an uncomfortable ordeal; the introduction of a vaginal speculum can be painful. The doctor may need to use a small, narrow speculum usually used for examining young girls. Insertion of fingers or a penis during sexual activity can be equally uncomfortable. The vagina can become easily irritated and sore with any form of penetration. The thrusting of the penis inside an atrophied vagina can cause excessive friction and discomfort. Many women experience a mild burning sensation, or in more severe cases, even a tearing sensation during intercourse. A few patients have told me they felt their vaginal walls were being ripped apart. Some women may experience increased bladder irritability with intercourse and may need to urinate more frequently.

Loss of Sexual Desire

In many women, vaginal pain and discomfort due to atrophic changes can cause a loss of sexual desire. Until the problem is treated and solved, these women, not surprisingly, try to avoid sex. Even women who formerly enjoyed sex may make excuses or stay away from intimate situations in which they may feel compelled to engage in sexual activity. If the husband or partner wishes to maintain frequent episodes of lovemaking, lack of interest on the woman's part can create a great deal of stress in the relationship. (In other circumstances, I have seen stress occur when the woman is interested in sex and her partner isn't. Relationships tend to suffer when the sexual interests of both parties differ greatly.)

In addition to the physical changes that make sexual activity uncomfortable, lack of hormonal support also decreases sexual arousal and sexual desire. Many postmenopausal women report a decrease in frequency and intensity of orgasm. Clitoral sensitivity can decline, as does the sensitivity of the cervix to a deep thrusting of the penis. Women may find their enjoyment of sex greatly diminished after menopause. As a result, frequency of sexual intercourse may decrease to less than once a month. Many of these physical changes are due to decreased estrogen stimulation of the nerve cells and blood vessels. Both nerve cells and blood vessels contain high levels of estrogen receptors. Lack of estrogen causes poor circulation to the genital region and decreased nerve response during sexual intercourse (or any sexual activity).

The availability of testosterone also has a very strong effect on sexual desire or libido. Testosterone is produced during our active reproductive years by both the ovaries and the adrenals. Ten to twenty percent of women experience a drop in libido soon after ceasing menstruation; this is because their ovaries stop making testosterone as well as estrogen. In other women, the drop in testosterone may not occur until some years after menopause. As a result, their sexual desire may not decrease as rapidly and their libido may stay intact for some years. In fact, some women (approximately 10 percent) report an increase in libido after menopause.

Some women find the lack of fear about becoming pregnant and the absence of menstruation quite liberating; they enjoy the increased sexual freedom without having to worry about birth control. Some women (and men) find that the increased privacy that occurs when children leave home (which can occur prior to, or around, the time of menopause) brings more sexual enjoyment, frequency and spontaneity in a home now shared primarily by the couple.

Vaginal and Bladder Infections

Vaginal infections can occur frequently in postmenopausal women because of the thinning and drying of the vaginal lining. The lining becomes easily irritated and injured, and as a result, it becomes very susceptible to infections by unhealthy organisms such as yeast and bacteria. The lack of estrogen support also causes the vaginal pH to change from acidic to alkaline. Healthy organisms such as lactobacillus thrive in an acidic environment, while the growth of harmful fungi and bacteria is inhibited.

When the pH becomes too alkaline, the reverse occurs. Our normal healthy bacteria die off and are replaced by organisms that thrive in an alkaline pH. These organisms infect the tissues and cause uncomfortable symptoms such as vaginal discharge, burning, and unpleasant odor. These infections may be difficult to eradicate and may recur frequently even after treatment. Many women develop symptoms every time they have sexual intercourse. This occurs because the trauma to the fragile tissues caused by penile penetration make the environment attractive to harmful pathological organisms.

Recurrent urinary tract infections can also be a difficult and unpleasant problem for many postmenopausal women. Standard medical textbooks state that 10 percent of these women suffer from recurrent infections and that the incidence of urine contaminated by unhealthy bacteria (without causing symptoms) is 25 percent. In fact, an estimated 10 to 15 percent of women over age 60 have frequent urinary tract infections.

Why do so many urinary tract infections occur? First, with the loss of estrogen support, the urethra, a small tube near the vaginal opening through which urine leaves the body, becomes less flexible and elastic. Like the vagina, the walls of the urethra thin out and become drier with time. Because the urethra is located so near the vaginal opening, it can become easily irritated after sexual intercourse and is more prone to infection. However, urinary tract infections are common even in women who aren't sexually active.

Other factors also play a role in this process. As women age, the lower urinary tract stops manufacturing anti-adherence factors which help prevent bacteria from attaching to the bladder wall. Common symptoms of urinary tract infection include urinary frequency, burning and itching. Women may have to urinate often but void only a small amount of urine. Occasionally, the infection travels from the urethra and bladder up to the kidneys and causes a severe infection that can require hospitalization.

Stress Incontinence

Estrogen helps maintain muscle tone and firmness. When the estrogen supply dwindles, the uterus, vagina and bladder can lose their tone; the ligaments that help support these organs also lose their tone. As a result, the bladder, rectum and uterus can drop or prolapse. If the bladder prolapses, it can bulge or pouch into the vagina; this condition is called a cystocele. When the bladder is involved, women may suffer from incontinence or an inability to control their flow of urine. They may leak urine when they laugh, cough or sneeze. Sometimes the loss of urine is enough to soil undergarments and women may need to wear a small pad. When the rectum bulges into the vagina, it is called a rectocele. Women with a rectocele may complain of constipation. When the uterus prolapses, women may have a sensation of fullness or heaviness in their pelvis because the uterus has dropped and is not suspended in its normal position.

Therapies for Relief of Vaginal and Bladder Aging

While nutritional and hormonal therapies are discussed later on in this book, I do want to discuss several categories of treatment that may result in the desired symptom relief for women suffering from atrophic changes. These include lubricants, physical activity including Kegel exercises, frequent sexual activity, and other supportive therapy.

Lubricants

The many excellent water-based lubricants currently on the market provide additional moisture for both partners. When used vaginally or rubbed on the penis, it can reduce the friction and discomfort of sexual intercourse if the tissues tend to be dry. Good products include Astroglide (Bio Film, Inc.)—a favorite with many of my patients—and K-Y Jelly (Johnson & Johnson), which can be squeezed from a tube or bottle. Some women prefer to use a newer product called Replens (Parke-Davis) which is a moisturizing gel inserted as a suppository; each application of Replens lasts for three days. It acts by plumping up the cells of the vaginal lining with moisture. In addition, Replens has an acidic pH that helps to protect against vaginal infections by discouraging the growth of unhealthy organisms.

Other women prefer to use massage oil, vitamin E liquid, or suppositories for additional lubrication. Although both of these can be quite helpful, it is important to avoid vaginal use of other oil-based products, such as Vaseline or baby oil. Unlike vitamin E and massage oil, which are vegetable oil based, these petroleum-based products will coat the vaginal lining and inhibit the release of your own secretions. They can even put women at higher risk of vaginal infections. Products designed for vaginal lubrication are safer and more effective for regular use.

Pelvic Activity

As mentioned earlier, regular sexual activity promotes better blood circulation to the vagina, as well as better tone and elasticity of the pelvic muscles and increased lubrication. Sexual activity stimulates all aspects of pelvic health if engaged in at least once or twice a week.

Local exercises of the pelvic area can improve bladder control and vaginal elasticity, even increasing sexual pleasure. Dr. Arnold Kegel developed a set of exercises in the 1940s that all women should practice during the menopausal years. The Kegel exercises strengthen the muscles that surround the urethra, vagina, and anus. Women who do these exercises frequently find that they are more aware of their vagina, find sex more pleasurable and they report more sensation in the pelvic area. Women also notice less leaking of urine when they cough, sneeze or laugh.

The Kegel exercises are simple and easy to do; they can be done any-where—sitting, standing or lying down. To practice these exercises:

- Draw up the vaginal muscles, hold for three seconds, and then relax. Repeat ten times.
- Squeeze your vaginal muscles firmly, then alternately contract and relax the muscles as rapidly as you can. Repeat ten times.

Preventive Suggestions for Vaginal Infections

To prevent vaginal infections (vaginitis), you may find it helpful to use an acidophilus supplement to help colonize your intestinal tract and vagina with the helpful bacteria that thrive in an acid environment. Nondairy yogurt with live acidophilus cultures is available in most health food stores. Nondairy yogurt is made of soybeans, almond or coconut and is an excellent food for menopausal women.

Don't binge on sugar, chocolate, or alcohol, which can promote the overgrowth of candida and trigger vaginal yeast infections. Avoid local irritation by washing with non-perfumed soap and water. After a bowel movement, wipe from front to back to avoid contamination of the vaginal and urethral tissues by intestinal bacteria. Do not wear panty hose and clothes that are tight in the crotch area as these can irritate fragile tissues. Wear cotton undergarments instead of synthetic material, which does not allow for proper drainage or air circulation in the crotch area.

If an infection is developing or if you are prone to infections, douche gently with one to two tablespoons of white vinegar in a quart of warm water. Some women find that vitamin C helps prevent vaginal infections from developing.

Be aware when selecting your sexual partner that sexually transmitted diseases (STDs) are more prevalent than ever before, and more dangerous. A partner who has had sex with many other women is much more likely to be harboring an organism that can give you an infection. If you are concerned about this issue, or in fact, if you are in any relationship that has not been totally monogamous for the past several years, ask your partner to wear a condom.

Preventive Suggestions for Urinary Tract Infections

Good hygiene also helps prevent urinary tract infections. Be sure to wash daily using a non-perfumed or nonirritating soap and warm water and urinate several times a day. Holding your urine increases the chance of developing an infection. Drink plenty of water, at least eight glasses a day. Urinating more frequently prevents your urine from becoming very concentrated and helps flush out your bladder. Urinate immediately before and after sexual intercourse. Many women are more prone to both vaginal and urinary tract infections after sexual activity.

Many books recommend the use of acidifying agents like cranberry juice to prevent infections. However, some studies have found that doing the reverse, or alkalinizing the urinary tract with 1/4 to 1/2 teaspoon of sodium bicarbonate (baking soda) or sodium citrate several times a day, is more effective in reducing pain, burning, and frequency of recurrence in women who are prone to bladder infections. Also, an alkaline form of vitamin C (the acidity of which is reduced through the addition of minerals). As previously mentioned, nondairy yogurt with live acidophilus culture is a delicious and healthy food. Unfortunately, it is not available in most supermarkets, but can be found in many health food stores.

Symptoms of Vaginal and Bladder Aging

Vaginal soreness and painful intercourse

Loss of sexual desire

Vaginal and bladder infections

Stress incontinence

Therapies for Relief of Vaginal and Bladder Aging

Estrogen Replacement Therapy (ERT)

Estrogen oral tablets, transdermal patch or vaginal cream

Testosterone tablets or cream

Lubricants

Pelvic activity

Sexual activity

Kegel exercises

5

Menopausal Mood Swings

During the menopause years, women may notice that their moods fluctuate more easily. Mood changes can vary from increased anxiety and irritability to depression and fatigue. Many women become distressed by these changes because they affect the quality of their personal relationships. Women report being bad tempered toward family, friends and co-workers and responding to daily life stresses in a more irritable fashion.

Many women describe these feelings as similar to the emotional ups and downs of premenstrual syndrome (PMS). A woman who has had PMS during her active reproductive years may be particularly distressed by her emotional fluctuations. Often, the expectation is that PMS symptoms will stop, rather than exacerbate, during the transition into menopause.

Luckily, not every woman experiences such pronounced emotional swings (in fact, some women go through menopause with no mood changes at all). However, if you are among those women who do, you will find very helpful information in this chapter on the causes of, and treatments for, menopausal mood swings.

Causes of Mood Swings are Complex

The complex causes of mood swings in most women can be due to hormonal changes, social and cultural factors, or more commonly, a combination of both. Some women are very sensitive to the rapid drop in their estrogen and progesterone levels that occurs with menopause. They may feel as if they are on an emotional roller coaster as their hormones drop and readjust to a new, lower level.

This is because estrogen and progesterone have a profound effect on the mood as well as the body. Progesterone has a sedative effect on the nervous system. When levels are too high, women may feel depressed and tired. On the other hand, estrogen has a stimulant effect on the nervous system, causing anxiety and irritability when estrogen output is elevated. Conversely, women may feel more depressed and moody when estrogen levels are diminished.

Under optimal conditions, estrogen output and progesterone output exist in a state of healthy equilibrium in the body. When you feel emotionally comfortable and you are not experiencing extreme mood fluctuations, these hormones are probably in balance. However, with the transition into menopause, hormonal levels shift rapidly, fluctuating between very high and low levels, then occasionally settling into balance again. Finally, both hormones drop permanently to low, postmenopausal levels. Likewise, moods may follow no obvious pattern, fluctuating as the hormones shift in sensitive women.

Unstable hormone levels can also affect how well we handle our daily life stresses. Research studies suggest that estrogen affects catecholamine levels in the body. Catecholamines are chemicals that affect the sympathetic nervous system. (This is the part of our nervous system that governs our "fight-or-flight" response or how our body deals with stress.) When the sympathetic nervous system is triggered, it causes muscles to tense, blood vessels to constrict, and heart and pulse rate to speed up to prepare for reacting to an emergency.

Women in early menopause may find the fight-or-flight response more easily triggered in response to day-to-day stress. This may put them in a frequent state of tension. They tend to react to small stresses the same way they would react to emergencies. The energy that accumulates in the body to meet this "emergency" must then be discharged. Women may become upset and angry before, once again, the system comes into balance.

For women, the social and cultural factors occurring before, during and after menopause may be quite stressful and can contribute to their mood fluctuations. For some women, menopause may signal loss of reproductive function, which may be experienced as a loss. For other women, menopause is a time when children leave home and move away, major career changes are made or a marriage ends in divorce.

The combination of hormonal and biochemical changes, plus lifestyle changes, can be quite difficult for many women to handle. Some women find themselves alone without their old familiar support systems intact during this time of transition. Other women find they have to cope with a husband's midlife crisis, engendered by loss of job or job dissatisfaction, health problems and other issues that are common for men around midlife. Some women become emotionally distressed at the bodily changes that menopause causes. Many women mention feeling unhappy with the wrinkles, loss of muscle tone and change in body shape that can occur very rapidly after menopause.

Solutions for Menopausal Mood Swings

Menopause-related mood swings can be relieved through a variety of therapeutic approaches. These include the use of HRT, mood-altering medications, counseling and support groups, and a variety of self-help methods. The first three of these methods are discussed in this chapter. More specific information on self-help methods is presented in the alternative therapy part of this book.

6

Osteoporosis & Other Physical Changes

One of the most serious consequences of postmenopausal aging is the development of osteoporosis. In fact, osteoporosis is a major health problem affecting more than 25 million older Americans, 90 percent of them women. One out of three American women will develop osteoporosis, most after menopause. A recent study reported in *The Endocrinologist* stated that the total medical costs related to osteoporosis exceed $10 billion annually.

The statistics surrounding osteoporosis are astounding. More than 1.3 million fractures occur each year as a result of this condition. Eighty percent of the 250,000 hip fractures in the United States each year occur in women over age 65 as a result of osteoporosis. About one-quarter of these women die within one year from complications, such as blood clots and pneumonia, caused by their convalescence.

Another one-third never regains the ability to function physically or socially on their own. These women spend the rest of their lives requiring long-term care in nursing facilities. In addition to causing hip fractures, osteoporosis is also responsible for loss of bone in the jaw, gum recession, dowager's hump, loss of height, back pain due to compression and fractures of the vertebra, and fractures of the wrist.

Often these fractures occur when only mild stress is put on the bone. This can include missing a step and falling down, falling on an extended arm or lifting a heavy object. Because of the underlying weakness of the bone, fractures can also occur spontaneously without any preceding trauma. This often occurs with vertebral fractures.

This chapter will discuss what happens to bones with osteoporosis, risk factors for osteoporosis, diagnosis of osteoporosis and other structural changes associated with menopause. Finally, therapies for osteoporosis and other structural changes will be explored.

What Happens to Bones with Osteoporosis

Bones are living tissue; we are constantly forming new bone cells to add to our skeletal mass and removing old cells that are no longer useful. This simultaneous addition and subtraction of bone from our skeleton is called bone remodeling. Between five to ten percent of our bone is replaced through this process every year. Bone remodeling involves two types of bone cells. Osteoblasts create new bone cells, while osteoclasts are responsible for removing old cells from the skeleton. This delicately balanced process is carefully regulated by many of the hormones in our body such as estrogen, progesterone, calcitonin and thyroid (as well as other hormones).

During the first 30 to 35 years of life, we deposit more bone in our skeleton than we lose, provided our health status is normal. In fact, our bone mass is at its peak in our 20s and begins to decrease in the mid-30s. According to peak bone mass theory, our bones reach their peak level of healthy density by the early 20s. The healthier our bones are at this stage, the less risk of osteoporosis later in life.

In the years preceding menopause, bone loss begins to exceed the addition of new bone to the skeleton. As a result, bones begin to lose important minerals such as calcium, as well as their matrix or intracellular substance. This causes a decrease in bone density as well as an increased brittleness or porousness of the bones.

Initially, this process occurs very slowly, and women are not even aware that it is going on. However, with loss of hormonal support to the bones at the time of menopause, this process accelerates. The first years after the onset of menopause can be a time of rapid bone loss for many women unless they have instituted therapies that emphasize prevention. Bone is lost at the rate of one to three percent per year for five to ten years after menopause. If the process of bone loss continues unabated, osteoporosis may eventually result.

Unfortunately, most women are unaware that they are losing bone during their early postmenopausal years. By the time osteoporosis becomes apparent as they begin to suffer from pain and fractures, women are already in their 60s or 70s. Older women with osteoporosis may have lost as much as 40 to 45 percent of their total bone mass.

Men also start to lose bone mass around age 40 (approximately three to five percent per decade). However, they have thicker bones to start with; men have approximately 30 percent more bone mass than women. In addition, the male hormone, testosterone, helps maintain bone mass and strength. Both estrogen in women and testosterone in men help control calcium absorption by the bones. These hormones prevent the reabsorption of calcium from the bones into the blood circulation where calcium can be excreted from the body.

However, unlike women whose estrogen levels drop precipitously at menopause, men can maintain their testosterone levels well into old age. As a result, their bones remain thicker and stronger far longer than those of women. This translates into more osteoporosis-related fractures for women than men—eight times more hip fractures and ten times more wrist fractures.

Although gender and age contribute greatly to the fractures that occur in old age because of osteoporosis, these are not the only factors. Many physicians also attribute fractures in the elderly to poor balance and lack of ability to right oneself when tripping or stumbling. Many older people lack flexibility, so when they fall, they absorb a much greater shock than if they could cushion themselves effectively or right themselves quickly. As a result, hip fractures increase with age, mirroring the loss of agility that occurs for many elderly women (and men).

Risk Factors for Osteoporosis

Not all women have the same risk of developing osteoporosis. Some women maintain strong and heavy bones throughout their lives, while other women develop accelerated bone loss soon after menopause. If you suspect you are at risk of developing osteoporosis, become knowledgeable about which factors have been linked to a higher incidence of this disease. This will help you and your physician evaluate your risk when planning an optimal treatment program. These factors include racial background, family history, hormonal status, lifestyle habits and pre-existing health conditions.

Racial Background

Skin pigmentation appears to parallel bone mass. African-American women are less likely to develop osteoporosis than Caucasian women. In fact, women at the highest risk are small and fair-skinned. These are typically women of Northern European ancestry such as Dutch, German or English background with blond, reddish or light brown hair and pale skin. Asian women have a higher risk of developing osteoporosis, too. Even among similar groups, the risk is lower with women who have darker skin. For example, in Israel the darker skin Sephardic Jews have a lower rate of fractures than do Jewish women of European origin.

Family History

If your close female relatives suffered from osteoporosis, you have a higher risk of developing this problem. Many women have seen their mothers or grandmothers develop a dowager's hump or become disabled after suffering a hip fracture. This can be quite upsetting for the entire family who must deal with the long-term disability.

Hormonal Status

The age at which women begin menopause and how much hormonal support they maintain during their postmenopausal years affects bone density. Women who have had a surgical menopause before age 40 with removal of their ovaries are at high risk of osteoporosis because of the abrupt withdrawal of estrogen at a young age. Similarly, women who go through an early natural menopause are at high risk. A woman going through early menopause at age 35 or 40 has as much as 10 to 15 years less estrogen protection for her bones than a woman going through menopause at age 50. Thus, the older you are when going through menopause, the more years of hormonal protection are provided for your bones.

Although obesity is a health risk for many diseases such as osteoarthritis and uterine cancer, being overweight does offer some protection against osteoporosis in postmenopausal women. This is because the fat cells produce a type of estrogen called estrone through conversion of an adrenal hormone called androstenedione. This type of estrogen provides some support for the bones once the ovarian source of estrogen has dwindled.

Lifestyle Habits

Women who engage in regular physical exercise and are more muscular have a lower risk of developing osteoporosis. Physical activity also helps keep women flexible and agile which reduces the likelihood of fractures. Conversely, inactivity increases your risk. Young women and men confined to bed for long periods show a decrease in bone mass.

Many nutritional factors affect your risk of developing osteoporosis, too. Women who drink more than two cups of coffee per day or large amounts of other caffeine-containing beverages such as black tea or colas, or who consume more than two alcoholic drinks per day, are at higher risk. Smokers also run a higher risk of osteoporosis. High protein or salt intake are risk factors, as is inadequate calcium intake. When you do not have an adequate intake of calcium, the body takes it from your bones to maintain a blood level necessary for various processes such as heart rhythm and blood clotting.

Pre-Existing Health Issues

Women with a history of bulimia, anorexia or malabsorption syndrome have an increased risk of poor calcium absorption or low estrogen levels (often the case in women with anorexia who do not have a body fat level high enough to produce adequate estrogen). Women who use thyroid medication, suffer from an overactive thyroid gland, or use cortisone for a variety of chronic conditions are at higher risk. This is also true of women with chronic kidney disease. All these conditions can adversely affect calcium balance in the body.

Risk Factors for Osteoporosis

Membership in a nonblack ethnic group

Fair, pale skin color

Having female relatives with osteoporosis

Early menopause (before age 40)

Being short and thin

Childlessness

High alcohol use (more than 5 ounces per day)

High caffeine use

Smoking

Low calcium diet

Lack of vitamin D

High-salt diet

High-protein diet

Chronic diarrhea or surgical removal of stomach or small intestine

Lactose deficiency

Daily use of cortisone

Use of thyroid medication (over 2 grains), Dilantin, or aluminum-containing antacids

Uremia (kidney disease)

Diagnosis of Osteoporosis

If you are not sure about the status of your bones, excellent tests are available to evaluate the likelihood of developing osteoporosis. The tests also allow physicians to diagnose osteoporosis in the early stages before the bone loss is so severe that fractures occur. These tests include the single-photon densitometer, which measures the density of the forearm; dual photon densitometer, which measures the spine or hip bone; and computerized axial tomography (also called a CAT scan), which can measure bone density in the spine. The CAT scan uses higher x-ray dosages and is a more expensive test. These tests are much more sensitive than conventional x-ray, which picks up osteoporosis only when 30 percent or more of the bone mass is lost.

You may choose to have a bone density test done if you are trying to decide whether or not to use HRT. If the tests show accelerated bone loss for your age group, you should seriously consider the use of HRT unless other major health issues contraindicate the use of hormones.

Another test for osteoporosis involves collecting a 24-hour urine sample. The laboratory then determines the ratio in the urine of calcium to a chemical called creatinine. A high calcium ratio indicates increased calcium excretion and accelerated bone loss.

Other Structural Changes Associated With Menopause

The loss of hormonal support affects not only the bones and teeth but also other structural elements of the body such as the joints, muscles, body shape, skin and hair. Although bone loss may occur silently for many years, the changes become more apparent within a few years of entering menopause.

For instance, the incidence of osteoarthritis increases, or women who have never experienced joint pain suddenly become symptomatic. Women with pre-existing arthritis often find that their symptoms get worse. Increased stiffness in the hands and shoulders as well as low back pain are common complaints. The hormonal link to osteoporosis was confirmed in a study reported in the *Annals of Rheumatic Diseases*. This study followed 606 women, aged 45 to 64, who used HRT for more than twelve months. A three-fold reduction in the incidence of osteoporosis of the knee was found in contrast to women who had never taken hormones or who had stopped their use two years prior to the study.

The lack of sex hormones also affects muscle tone throughout the body after menopause, including sagging of the breast, facial, and arm muscles, as well as the loss of pelvic muscle tone which can affect sexual pleasure and the ability to hold urine. The lack of estrogen is probably also responsible for the increase in low back and pelvic pain that women experience around this time.

Another visible sign of aging for many women after menopause is a change in body shape as the distribution of weight on the body changes.

The waist and upper back get thicker, while the hips and breasts tend to lose some of their fat. The result is that the female shape changes from an hourglass figure to a pear shape. Many women find that not only does their figure shape change, but they also gain weight more easily (10 to 15 pounds in the year or two following menopause isn't unusual). This can occur no matter how diligently they diet or how much they exercise.

The lack of female hormonal support plus the slowing of the metabolism are probably responsible for these changes. Women after menopause don't burn calories as efficiently as during their younger years. Careful attention to diet and regular exercise can certainly help, but may not entirely correct, these physical changes. I recommend that you read the alternative therapy chapters in this book for more in-depth information.

The skin and hair undergo many changes after menopause due to loss of estrogen. There is a gradual tendency toward thinning and dryness of the skin. Skin pigmentation becomes uneven which affects coloration. Some women may lose their even skin tone and notice patches of lighter and darker skin.

As collagen production in the skin slows down, the skin loses its elasticity. The underlying muscle and fat tissues that help give skin its underlying support begins to shrink. There is also a reduction in sweat gland activity and decreased tolerance to temperature changes. As a result, many visible signs of skin aging become apparent such as pronounced wrinkling and creasing. Many women find these changes cosmetically unappealing and employ a variety of dermatologic aids in an attempt to make their skin look younger and healthier.

Women who smoke, have poor nutritional habits or have had excessive exposure to sunlight are more likely to show signs of skin aging at a younger age. Conversely, women who tend to carry a little extra weight or have reached menopause at a later age will have better-looking skin. This is because they have had higher circulating levels of estrogen in their bodies for more years than a thin woman who enters menopause at an early age.

Lack of estrogen also affects the hair. With menopause, hair on the head and in the pubic area becomes drier, coarser and sparser. Women may also notice the growth of darker or coarser hair in areas where they've never had hair before, such as the chin, upper lip, chest or abdomen. This unusual growth of hair is due to the stimulation of the hair follicle by low amounts of androgens, a type of male hormone.

High estrogen levels block the action of these male hormones on hair follicle receptors. However, after menopause, these low amounts of androgen may not decrease to the same extent that estrogen does in certain women. These unopposed androgens can then affect the pattern of hair growth and hair loss, taking on a more male like pattern.

Other Supportive Measures

While many supportive measures are mentioned in the alternative therapy section of this book, there are many actions a woman can take to prevent damage to her bones, joints, muscles, skin and hair after menopause. Healthy lifestyle habits can slow down the aging of all these bones and tissues. These beneficial measures include the following.

- Do regular weight-bearing exercise, such as walking or weight training, at least thirty minutes per day. This helps keep bones strong and intact and promotes good blood circulation.

- Practice stretching exercises to keep your joints and muscles limber and flexible.

- Limit cigarette use and alcohol intake.

- Avoid sun exposure unless you use a high SPF sunscreen (15 or more). The sun causes damage and aging of the skin if protection from its rays is not used regularly.

- Drink lots of water—at least eight glasses per day—to thoroughly hydrate your skin and other tissues.

- Apply moisturizers to your skin to help lock in the fluid.

- Lose weight slowly if you diet. Rapid weight loss can accelerate the aging of your skin's appearance.

- Avoid over processing your hair with permanents and other hair care techniques that can cause excessive dryness and splitting of the hair.

- If you want to have unwanted hair removed, consider electrolysis. This is the only permanent method for hair removal. It is important, however, to work with an experienced and knowledgeable operator.

- Follow the dietary and nutritional recommendations for healthy bones, skin, muscles and joints discussed in this book.

Structural Components of the Body that Show Menopausal Changes

Bones

Joints

Muscles

Skin

Hair

7

Heart Disease and Stroke

Coronary heart disease is the main killer of American women, claiming the lives of more than a quarter of a million women per year. More women die from heart disease than die from all forms of cancer. Although younger women also die of heart disease, it occurs less frequently during the active reproductive years. The incidence of heart disease escalates as women age. From age 30 to 60, cancer is the main cause of death in women, with heart disease in second place from age 40 to 60. Over age 60, heart disease becomes the leading cause of death in women.

Most women die from heart attacks due to coronary artery disease, where there is a narrowing of one or more of the arteries that supply blood and oxygen to the heart. This narrowing is caused by the formation of plaque in the arteries. Plaque is a thick, waxy, yellowish substance consisting primarily of cholesterol, smooth muscle cells and foam cells.

As the formation of plaque progresses, it can obstruct the flow of blood through the blood vessels. Over time, this will seriously compromise function of the heart, finally leading to a heart attack. Unfortunately, the obstruction is usually quite advanced before it begins to cause symptoms of chest pain, angina and shortness of breath on mild exertion.

General Risk Factors for Heart Disease

Extensive research has been done over the past few decades to determine if certain women run a higher risk of developing heart disease. A number of interesting medical studies have focused on a variety of factors that appear linked to the likelihood of developing heart disease. These include specific physical characteristics, family history, blood lipid profile, hypertension, diabetes, as well as lifestyle factors such as diet, smoking, lack of activity and stress.

Physical Characteristics

Age. As mentioned earlier, the older the woman, the greater her risk of developing heart disease. The highest incidence is in women older than age 65.

Body Weight. Women weighing 20 to 30 percent over their ideal weight are considered to be at greater risk of developing heart disease. This was noted in an eight-year study by Harvard Medical School, which followed more than 115,000 women. Excess weight was found to be a significant factor in women developing coronary artery disease during the study period.

Body Shape—Distribution of Fat. Not only is overall obesity a risk factor but also how the fat is distributed on the body. Women with excess weight concentrated in the mid-section of their bodies, with a shape like an apple, have a higher risk of coronary artery disease than pear-shaped women, who distribute their fat to their hips and thighs.

Family History of Heart Disease. You are at higher risk of developing heart disease if close relatives have had a heart attack at an early age. Statistically, the risk increases if your father had a heart attack before age 56 or your mother before age 60. Similarly, you are at higher risk if any of your grandparents had a heart attack at a young age.

Blood Lipid Profile

Elevated Triglycerides. Elevated triglycerides are a type of fat consisting of three fatty acid molecules hooked to a glycerol backbone. Triglycerides are the form in which fat is stored in the body's tissues. Normal triglyceride levels range from 50 to 200 mg/dl. Triglycerides elevated in the blood to a level of 200 mg/dl or greater indicate a greater risk of developing coronary artery disease.

Elevated Total Cholesterol and LDL Cholesterol. Cholesterol is a yellowish, waxy substance manufactured in the body primarily by the liver and, to a lesser extent, by the intestines. We also ingest cholesterol in our diet when we eat dairy and meat products and fish. Cholesterol is needed for the synthesis of our sex hormones; it is the initial ingredient for sex hormone production. Cholesterol is also necessary for the synthesis of cell membranes and other essential body substances such as the sheath or coating of the nerves and bile.

How effectively cholesterol is used depends on its efficient transport throughout the body and how well the body can store or dispose of any excess. Transportation in the body is a potential problem because the fatty cholesterol isn't soluble in blood, which is mostly water. To solve this problem the body packages the cholesterol with a protein that allows the fat to be mixed with the blood. This process takes place in the liver where several types of cholesterol-protein mixtures are produced.

The major type of cholesterol-protein manufactured is low-density lipoprotein, or LDL, the body's main carrier of cholesterol. When LDL levels are elevated, it is believed to remain in the blood stream. The excessive levels of LDL are thought to injure the endothelium (the inner lining of the blood vessel wall), thereby initiating plaque formation. Thus, LDL is considered to be the "bad" type of cholesterol. Women with a total blood cholesterol above 200 mg/dl and a LDL level above 129-120 mg/dl are thought to be at higher risk of heart disease.

Decreased HDL Cholesterol. The liver makes another type of lipoprotein called high-density lipoprotein, or HDL, the "good" type of cholesterol. This is because HDL picks up and carries excess cholesterol back to the liver where it is secreted into the bile. The bile empties the excess cholesterol into the intestinal tract where it is excreted from the body through bowel movements. When the HDL is less than 50 mg/dl, a woman is considered to be at higher risk of coronary artery disease. When the HDL is above 60 mg/dl it is considered to confer a lower risk for women.

Elevated LDL to HDL Ratio. The ratio between the LDL and HDL is also an important indicator of heart disease risk. The LDL to HDL ratio of 4.4 signifies an average risk of heart disease, 3.3 ratio is about half average; while 7 is about double the risk.

C-reactive Protein (CRP). This is a protein produced within the liver and found in the blood. It is an important marker of inflammation. Patients with elevated levels of CRP have an increased risk of cardiovascular disease, hypertension, and diabetes.

Hypertension

High blood pressure is a significant risk factor for developing coronary artery disease. Sixty million Americans have elevated blood pressure readings. Nearly half of these are women. Blood pressure is considered to be elevated when the reading is above 140/90. The first number indicates the systolic pressure, the pressure that occurs when the heart contracts and pushes blood through the arterial circulation. The second number indicates the diastolic blood pressure, the pressure in the arteries when the heart relaxes between beats. Not only does hypertension increase the likelihood of heart attacks, but it also increases your risk of strokes and kidney disease.

Diabetes

The Framingham Heart Study, an important study of cardiovascular disease risk, found that women with diabetes have twice as high a risk of developing a heart attack as non-diabetic women. Diabetic women are also at higher risk of developing serious visual problems and kidney complications, as well as hypertension and higher cholesterol levels.

Lifestyle Factors

In the past few decades, research has indicated that lifestyle factors play a major role in the development of disease. Lifestyle patterns such as diet, smoking, obesity, sedentary behavior and high stress all contribute to a high-risk profile for heart disease and stroke.

Cigarette Smoking. Women smokers have an increased risk of heart attacks and strokes (as do men smokers). This is because smoking narrows the diameter of the blood vessels, impairing circulation. Smokers are also more likely to have higher levels of the bad LDL and lower levels of the good HDL.

Cigarette smoking is also considered a major cause of stroke, the third leading cause of death in the United States. Nicotine increases the heart rate, which in turn, raises the blood pressure. Hypertension can be a precursor to stroke.

Unfortunately, seventeen percent of all women smoke, and this percentage is not declining rapidly despite the great amount of public information on the health perils of smoking. Women smokers also enter menopause two to three years earlier than nonsmokers.

Physical Inactivity. Women with sedentary lifestyles have a three times higher risk of developing heart disease than women who are physically active. The heart is a muscle that needs to be exercised. Women who engage in aerobic exercise, such as walking at least three times a week for a half hour, have a lower resting heart rate, greater lung capacity, and an improved ability to handle stress.

Stress. Several studies suggest that severe stress is a risk factor in women for developing coronary artery disease. Unfortunately, women have not been studied as frequently as men. Many studies have been done on the Type A hard-driving, aggressive male personality. However, women with multiple home and work responsibilities are often as hard driving and stressed as men. This can, over time, predispose certain women to an increased risk of heart attack.

Diet. In 1989, the National Research Council reported evidence of a direct relationship between dietary fat intake and the risk of cardiovascular disease, cancer and stroke. You can limit your long term risk of developing these conditions by 20 percent if you limit your fats to 30 percent of your daily calories, keep saturated fats to less than 10 percent and keep cholesterol levels down.

Female-Related Risk Factors

Some risk factors for heart disease are particularly female and directly relate to menopause and hormone levels.

Menopausal Status. The risk of coronary artery disease increases two to three fold once a woman enters natural menopause. Research studies, including the Framingham Heart Study (which has been ongoing since 1949), have confirmed that premenopausal women with intact ovarian function enjoy significant protection against the development of heart attacks.

Surgical or Natural Menopause Before Age 45. Recent studies have shown that women who undergo a hysterectomy, with removal of their ovaries during the premenopausal years, have three times more risk of coronary artery disease than women who cease menstruating later. Similarly, a study of 122,000 nurses found that women who went through surgical menopause before age 35 have two to seven times the risk of heart attack; the risk is also higher in women who go through natural menopause at an early age. Estrogen appears to confer significant protection against heart attacks during a woman's active reproductive years. The longer a woman menstruates, the more years of estrogenic protection her vascular system enjoys.

Part II:
Bioidentical Hormone Therapies

8

Bioidentical Estrogen Therapy

The use of hormones after menopause is a recent innovation in human history. Relatively few women even survived the rigors of more primitive societies to face the issue of postmenopausal aging. How long a woman lived did not depend on sophisticated hormonal therapies synthesized in a laboratory, but rather, on a combination of good genes, familial longevity, a healthy lifestyle with adequate nutrition, balanced responses to stress and a balance of physical activity and rest. Only since the turn of the century have women begun to outlive their menopause transition and continue to thrive and be active so for several more decades.

Scientists first isolated estrogen and progesterone in the laboratory in their purified state during the 1920s. In the decades before this advance, physicians prescribed various formulations of the whole gland. Animal ovaries were powdered, pulverized and liquefied and then given by health care providers to women who had gone through surgical menopause or to those who suffered from menstrual cramps. Use of hormones remained limited throughout the 1930s and 1940s.

By the 1950s and 1960s, the benefits of estrogen in treating menopausal symptoms were understood and appreciated and its use became wide-spread. A number of books and articles were written during this era about estrogen's many benefits, both real and fancied. Many women benefited from the relief estrogen brought from unpleasant hot flashes, vaginal dryness, mood swings and other symptoms. Women were told that estrogen would even enhance their attractiveness and youthfulness. However, very little was understood or communicated to women about the risks of using estrogen.

The first adverse reports about estrogen therapy surfaced in 1975. Several research studies published that year linked postmenopausal women using estrogen with cancer of the lining of the uterus (also called the endometrium). In those studies, women who used estrogen were four to eight times more likely to develop this cancer. Fearful of cancer, postmenopausal women avoided estrogen in dramatic numbers, and physicians were equally hesitant about prescribing it. Subsequent research has shown that the addition of progesterone has a protective benefit in terms of preventing uterine cancer.

Most women who in menopause continue to be offered conventional estrogen replacement therapy (and often, synthetic progesterone therapy called "progestins") by their physicians or health care provider. For decades, this type of therapy was considered the "gold standard" of care for women suffering from menopause symptoms due to estrogen deficiency.

Yet, in the past ten to fifteen years, landmark research studies have conclusively started to prove the dangers of conventional estrogen replacement therapy (ERT) as well as combination therapy in which synthetic or animal forms of estrogen are combined with synthetic progesterone or progestins (HRT). The many studies that have followed in the past decade have continued to build the case against these types of therapies. I have been following this research intensively and have had strong concerns regarding physicians' continued persistence in using HRT.

As women are becoming more and more aware of this negative research on hormone replacement therapy, they are also becoming more concerned about using these therapies to support their low levels of estrogen. Their concerns have included fear that estrogen replacement therapy could intensify serious preexisting health problems such as bloating, weight gain, breast tenderness, anxiety or depression, heavy bleeding from uterine fibroid tumors, severe migraine headaches, or blood clotting problems. Other women, free from illness, fear that the long-term use of estrogen may accelerate the onset of a disease for which they are at risk, based on a strong family history like breast cancer or heart disease. Some of my patients have refused to use estrogen on a philosophical basis, preferring instead to pursue nondrug treatment options such as nutritional therapies and acupuncture.

Happily, for women needing more hormonal support to compensate for the lack of estrogen that they are producing with the onset of menopause, bioidentical estrogen therapy can be prescribed by your physician or health care provider. Biochemically identical hormones are molecularly identical to the hormones found in the human body. Moreover, they are produced in the laboratory from natural ingredients such as soy and wild yam, derived from plants, not horse urine. Since bioidentical hormones are biologically similar to the hormones your body produces, they do not appear to have the grave risks associated with conventional HRT.

As mentioned earlier in this book, estradiol is the main type of estrogen manufactured by the ovaries during our active reproductive years, and estrone is the primary type of estrogen that we produce by our ovaries and adrenal glands after menopause. Estriol, the weakest and probably safest type of natural estrogen, is a metabolite of the two more potent estrogens produced in our bodies.

Based on various animal and human studies, it appears that estriol is less likely to promote excessive tissue growth, and even helps prevent breast and endometrial cancers.

It can now be manufactured from plant-based sources such as soy and diascorea composita, the wild yam plant, and can be ordered by physicians through compounding pharmacies.

Many women are currently requesting estriol from their physicians because it effectively relieves menopausal symptoms and produces fewer side effects than the more potent hormones, estrone and estradiol. For example, estrone and estradiol are growth stimulants to estrogen-sensitive tissues such as the uterine lining and the breast. When unopposed by the growth-limiting effect of progesterone, estrone and estradiol have been linked to increased risk of uterine and breast cancer. In contrast, estriol is not a growth stimulant and its main effect is on the vaginal lining. Estriol is effective for the treatment of vaginal dryness, hot flashes, and mood swings. Unlike the more potent estrogens, it does not appear to be beneficial to the bones or heart.

Several human studies indicate that it may be the ratio of estriol to estradiol and estrone that is protective. Women with higher amounts of estriol in relation to the other hormones were less likely to develop cancer, perhaps because estriol attaches to estrogen receptors that might otherwise bind to much more potent forms of estrogen that more readily promote cell proliferation. And, unlike conventional HRT that may cause fluid retention, headaches, nausea, and the buildup of uterine tissue, estriol has few, if any, side effects.

One study published in the *Journal of the American Medical Association* found that estriol was particularly effective in treating vaginal atrophy, mood swings, and hot flashes. Researchers selected 52 symptomatic, postmenopausal women and separated them into four groups, giving each group either 2 mg, 4 mg, 6 mg, or 8 mg of estriol per day for six months. On average, women in every group experienced a decrease in their menopausal symptoms after one month of treatment. Furthermore, in three of the four groups, women who had ranked their symptoms as severe now felt that their symptoms were very mild.

Another study from *Alternative Medicine Review* found that estriol provides the protection of conventional HRT without the risks. Additionally, estriol was shown to ease menopausal symptoms, including hot flashes, insomnia, vaginal dryness, and urinary tract infections.

A study from Taiwan showed similar results. Researchers gave 20 menopausal patients, aged 44–62 years, 2 mg of estriol a day for two years. They found that estriol was significantly effective in easing menopausal symptoms (especially hot flashes and insomnia) in 86 percent of patients. Additionally, estriol did not cause proliferation of the uterine lining. This is great news for women at high risk for endometrial cancer, such as those who are significantly overweight.

Other studies have supported estriol's benefit in treating recurrent urinary tract infections. In a study from the *New England Journal of Medicine*, researchers looked at 93 postmenopausal women with a history of recurrent urinary tract infections. After four months of treatment, the patients using estriol needed to use significantly fewer antibiotics for their bladder infections during the course of the study. Additionally, 95 percent of those who received the estriol remained disease-free. The only side effects noted with the use of estriol have been occasional mild itching and irritation.

Early research also suggests estriol may offer some protection to your bones. One study in particular found that estriol significantly improved bone mineral density. Researchers divided 24 elderly women into two groups. The first group received 2 mg of estriol a day for six months, while the other received a placebo; both groups were given 1,000 mg of calcium chloride per day. They found the group who took estriol enjoyed an increase in bone mineral density, while the control group actually saw a decrease in bone density.

A similar study published in the *Journal of Obstetrics and Gynecology Research* found that menopausal women who received 2 mg of estriol a day for 50 weeks enjoyed a significantly slower breakdown of bone. This was most noticeable in women who had been in menopause for at least five years. Patients also reported an improvement in menopausal symptoms.

More importantly, researchers found that estriol did not stimulate the uterine lining, which translates to a reduced risk for uterine cancer. Plus, the fact that it attaches to estrogen receptors in your breast tissue means estriol may help to block the more potent, and therefore carcinogenic, estrogens like estradiol from attaching to these receptors.

> **Sharon's Story**
>
> Sharon, a 63-year-old woman, came to see me with worsening urinary incontinence, which was interfering with her ability to take long hikes she used to do at least two to three times a week in the hilly area near her home. She was also distressed by her diminished ability to handle stress.
>
> Sharon shared with me that she was reacting to her husband's bad moods and her grown children's family issues with much greater anxiety than she had in the past. She went on to tell me that her sleep was also being affected, and she was waking up much more frequently in the middle of the night. She also mentioned that she continued to have hot flashes on and off, which were more frequent when she felt particularly stressed.
>
> I suggested that she start using my hormonal restoration program immediately, which included among other things bioidentical estrogen, melatonin, and valerian root. After several weeks, Sharon was much calmer and more relaxed. She was sleeping better and was even able to reduce her urinary incontinence.

Using Biochemically Identical Estrogen

Estriol can be taken orally or used topically. If taken orally, I recommend using 2–4 mg daily, in capsule form. When used topically, I suggest applying one gram of the cream to your vagina every night for two to four weeks, then use twice a week for maintenance. Many women with vaginal or bladder symptoms may choose just to use the vaginal cream locally, limiting their total body exposure to estrogen. However, I recommend covering the urethral and outer genital area with a thin layer of the cream as well as applying it intravaginally during the first few weeks of use.

In addition to estrogen alone, some researchers advocate the use of estriol in combination with estradiol (bi-estrogen or bivalent) or with estradiol and estrone (tri-estrogen or trivalent). In these combinations, the amount of estriol is far greater than the other forms of estrogen. In the case of trivalent estrogen, the ratios are usually 80 percent estriol and just 10 percent each estradiol and estrone. These combinations are also highly effective, and have also been shown to reduce menopausal symptoms, improve bone density, and increase "good" HDL cholesterol.

Estriol and all biochemically identical estrogen have to be prescribed by your physician. I have found that physicians in my area will often prescribe estriol when asked to by their patients. Estriol is available at most compounding pharmacies, as well as a few mainstream pharmacies. I recommend the Women's International Pharmacy in Madison, Wisconsin, which sends estriol formulations to physicians throughout the U.S. You can find them online at womensinternational.com or by calling 800-279-5708.

9

Bioidentical Progesterone

Before the 1980s, all progesterone therapy had to be administered by injection in the doctor's office. The development of oral progesterone-like chemicals made this hormone much more readily available. Initially, a synthetic type of progesterone was combined with estrogen in birth control pills for younger women. Then progesterone's important role in preventing endometrial cancer in postmenopausal women on estrogen replacement therapy (ERT) was discovered in the 1970s. In one study, cited in a review article in the *American Family Physician*, 5,563 postmenopausal women were followed for nine years. In women using estrogen alone, the incidence of endometrial cancer was 390.6 cases per 100,000 women per year. In contrast, with combined estrogen and progesterone therapy, the incidence was only 99 cases per 100,000 women per year.

Not only does progesterone confer protection in women using estrogen replacement therapy, but it actually appears to protect against the development of endometrial cancer in all postmenopausal women. In the same study, women using no estrogen therapy at all were at higher risk than those on progesterone because of their own endogenous estrogen. These women developed 245.5 cases of endometrial cancer per 100,000 women per year. Not only has the rate of this cancer declined with the use of progesterone, but those women who develop it tend to do so at a later age. After this and other similar studies, progesterone therapy rapidly became part of the standard hormonal regimen for postmenopausal women who still had their uterus intact.

The progesterone used in replacement therapy today, whether described as synthetic or natural, is all produced by commercial laboratories. The terms natural and synthetic refer to the actual structure of the progesterone molecule. Progesterone that is natural has the same structure as the hormone the body produces.

In contrast, while synthetic progesterone has somewhat the same function as the progesterone produced by the body—but many negative side effects—its structure differs slightly. In the United States, most prescriptions are for the synthetic form, called a progestin. The most common progestin is Provera, or medroxyprogesterone.

I do not recommend the use of synthetic progesterone, because many women develop negative side effects such as fatigue, depression, mood changes, breast tenderness and enlargement, and headaches. I, instead, prefer to recommend natural, bioidentical progesterone for women suffering from menopause related symptoms and to balance the use of estrogen replacement therapy.

Natural, biochemically identical progesterone became available in the early 1980s, but initially only as a rectal or vaginal suppository. Although many women found the use of natural progesterone to be helpful, using it as a suppository was messy, since it tended to leak from the rectum or vagina. Progestin remained the preferred form because it was easy to take as a pill and was also more absorbable.

However, natural progesterone was subsequently developed in a micronized form (pulverized into tiny particles) that is readily absorbed and is taken orally. The prescription name of this form of oral, natural progesterone is Prometrium, and must be prescribed by your physician. It can also be used as a topical skin cream, transdermal spray, sublingual drops and suppositories, much of which can be purchased without a physician's prescription from health food stores or through the Internet.

Using Natural Progesterone

Women of all ages (from their 30s on up) are currently using natural progesterone cream, which is now available in many health food stores and does not require a doctor's prescription (although the other forms of natural progesterone do require a prescription). Natural progesterone can be taken in oral micronized form or as a skin cream, rectal or vaginal suppository, or sublingual drops. Be sure to check the label of any product that you buy to make sure it truly contains pharmaceutical-grade, natural progesterone in therapeutic doses.

Oral Micronized Progesterone

Initially, natural progesterone could not be taken orally because it was destroyed during digestion and never reached the bloodstream. However, a micronized form of progesterone is now available that is protected from destruction by stomach acid and enzymes and can be absorbed and used by the body.

One study published in the *British Medical Journal* followed 23 women for four months. Each woman received 300 mg of oral progesterone daily for two continuous months. Those women receiving treatment had a clear improvement in concentration. Similar increases in mental acuity and the ability to remain focused on a subject have also been found in premeno-pausal and postmenopausal women.

Research has shown that oral progesterone can also reduce blood pressure. In a study also published in the *British Medical Journal*, researchers gave postmenopausal women and older men 200, 400, or 600 mg of oral progesterone or a placebo every day for two weeks. Those taking the prog-esterone enjoyed a significant decrease in their systolic blood pressure (the top number), as compared to the placebo group. In fact, participants who took 600 mg lowered their systolic blood pressure by about 19.7 mm Hg and their diastolic blood pressure (the bottom number) by about 9.6 mm Hg.

In menopausal women, dosages of 100-200 mg of natural, oral progesterone (Prometrium) taken daily can be effective, although the dose can vary in either direction. You need these high doses, as 85-90 percent of the amount consumed will be metabolized by the liver soon after it has been ingested. Like the synthetic progestins, perimenopausal women should use oral micronized progesterone 10-13 days per month. If you are in menopause, most physicians recommend using it every day.

Skin Cream

Progesterone cream is applied to the skin and absorbed into the general circulation. Recent research has shown that it not only elevates progesterone levels, but it also elevates DHEA levels in the body. Because it is absorbed through the skin, it bypasses the liver, thereby escaping liver metabolism. Unlike the synthetic progestins, there are few side effects reported by its use and it is available without a prescription.

Medical research studies have been very positive. According to a randomized, double-blind, placebo-controlled study from *Obstetrics and Gynecology*, transdermal progesterone cream relieved menopausal vaso-motor symptoms.

Researchers tested 90 postmenopausal women who were within five years of menopause and had not used any hormones for at least 12 months prior to the study. The women were tested for follicle-stimulating hormone levels; bone mineral density of the lumbar spine and hip; cholesterol levels; LDL, HDL, and triglyceride levels, and thyroid-stimulating hormone levels. All of the tests were repeated after one year. During that time, each woman kept a log of the number and severity of hot flashes.

The women were divided into two groups. In the first group, 43 of the women used ¼ teaspoon (20 mg) of progesterone cream a day, regularly rotating the application on their arm, breasts, or thighs. The other 47 women used a placebo. Of the women using the progesterone cream, 83 percent enjoyed fewer hot flashes, as compared to just 19 percent in the placebo group.

This finding was also confirmed by a study reported in *Gynecological Endocrinology*. Researchers found that women using 40 mg of transdermal progesterone cream a day for one year reported a significant reduction in hot flashes.

Other studies have shown that progesterone creams are also just as effective in increasing progesterone levels and easing menopausal symptoms as oral progestins—but significantly safer. According to a study presented at the annual meeting of the *American Society for Clinical*

Pharmacology and Therapeutics, women given either natural progesterone cream or a synthetic oral progestin exhibited the same blood levels of the hormone.

A range of progesterone creams, available without a prescription, contain anywhere from less than 2 mg to more than 400 mg of the hormone per jar. Pro-Gest cream, which contains more than 400 mg in a container, is one of the better-known brands. The cream is applied to the skin and absorbed into the general circulation and reaches more body tissues than oral progesterone, which is first metabolized by the liver and converted into three different compounds.

A typical dosage of natural progesterone is 40 mg a day. A two-ounce jar should last for over one month. If you are perimenopausal, you should apply the cream from day 12 to day 26 of your menstrual cycle. If you are menopausal and not taking estrogen, you may use progesterone for two to three weeks each month, though some physicians do recommend daily use to avoid withdrawal bleeding.

If you are self-medicating with progesterone cream in an effort to block the cancer-promoting effect of estrogen on the uterus, you need to make sure you are taking enough progesterone for it to be protective. Blood or saliva testing of progesterone levels will help to determine if the level of supplemental progesterone you're using is in the therapeutic range.

The cream is used twice daily in ¼ - ½ teaspoon amounts, generally upon rising in the morning and before going to bed at night. The cream can be applied to any area of the skin. Many women rub it into their chest, abdomen, arms, or back. If the cream is absorbed rapidly (under two minutes), it means that the body needs a higher dose, and a slightly higher amount may be used.

Note: Some reputed progesterone creams that contain wild yam extract contain only the precursor compound— diosgenin— and little to no progesterone. Also, progesterone delivered as a cream must suspend the hormone in a proper medium or it will not be effective.

A cream containing mineral oil will not allow the progesterone to be absorbed properly. Some products have not stabilized the progesterone and, as a result, the hormone deteriorates over time.

Laboratory testing, such as the saliva tests, of progesterone levels within the body can be used to determine the proper dosage. Progesterone cream is more likely to be prescribed by physicians knowledgeable about alternative therapies. Many physicians prescribe it for menopause symptoms and for the treatment of osteoporosis.

Helga's Story

I have worked with patients with decreased bone density, but who have refused conventional estrogen/progestin therapy. One such woman, Helga chose instead to use natural progesterone cream, along with a variety of dietary and plant-based estrogens, as well as a high-potency nutritional supplement that contained critical vitamins and minerals for bone health. She also adopted a vegetarian-based diet and started performing resistance exercises with weights.

Although she had a higher than normal risk of osteoporosis, given a 25 percent loss of bone mass by age 50, she showed a steady improvement in her bone density in the years after initiating my program.

Transdermal Sprays

Transdermal sprays work much like the creams, but without the mess. They are also quickly and efficiently absorbed into the skin with little need for rubbing. The spray also has a unique delivery system that makes it easier to absorb than the cream.

A typical dosage of the spray is 5 to 10 sprays per day, usually upon rising in the morning and before going to bed at night. Like the cream, the spray can be applied to any area of the skin. I find that most women prefer to spray it on their arms, thighs, or abdomen. I am particularly partial to the ProgestEase brand of progesterone spray.

Sublingual Drops

Progesterone is available in a vitamin E oil base. This is held under the tongue for at least one minute so that it is absorbed, rather than swallowed. This results in a quick rise in hormone levels, followed by a drop three to four hours later. It is necessary to take the drops three to four times a day to maintain stable blood levels.

Suppositories

Progesterone can also be taken as a rectal or vaginal suppository. Vaginal suppositories allow for excellent local intake of progesterone into the uterus, and may be helpful for pre- or perimenopausal women with heavy and irregular bleeding.

In a study published in the *Journal of Assisted Reproduction and Genetics*, twenty-five women with severe PMS and seventeen reproductive-age females participated in a controlled trial. Treatment consisted of a 200 mg vaginal progesterone suppository, taken twice daily. The researchers observed that the women receiving the progesterone reported significant improvement in mood symptoms and nervousness.

A randomized, double-blind, placebo-controlled study published in *American Journal of Obstetrics and Gynecology* also found that the use of a vaginal progesterone suppository reduced the risk of preterm labor. Researchers gave 142 high-risk pregnant women either 100 mg of progesterone a day (administered by vaginal suppository) or a placebo. All were monitored for uterine contraction once a week for 60 minutes, between weeks 24 and 34 of gestation. They found that those women taking the progesterone had less uterine contractions than those receiving the placebo. They also found that less than 14 percent of the women in the progesterone group delivered early, and less than three percent delivered before 34 weeks, as compared to more than 18 percent of the placebo group delivering before 34 weeks. Researchers concluded that progesterone suppositories reduce the frequency of uterine contractions and the threat of preterm delivery in high-risk women.

Benefits of Progesterone Therapy

Although progesterone is prescribed by gynecologists for other reasons than estrogen replacement therapy, it is still an important therapy for menopausal women. The major indications for use of progesterone are as follows: prevention of endometrial cancer, reduction of hot flashes, and prevention or treatment of osteoporosis. There are also other benefits when using natural progesterone, which I mention in this section.

Prevents Endometrial Cancer. As discussed earlier, prevention of endometrial cancer is the primary reason why physicians prescribe progesterone. Without the addition of progesterone to an estrogen treatment regimen, the incidence of endometrial cancer increases four to eight-fold in women with an intact uterus. The importance of progesterone therapy has been emphasized in a number of significant medical studies. In one study published in the *American Family Physician*, 5,563 postmenopausal women were followed for nine years. In women using estrogen alone, the incidence of endometrial cancer was 390.6 cases per 100,000 women per year. In contrast, with combined estrogen and progesterone therapy, the incidence was only 99 cases per 100,000 women per year. Not only does progesterone confer protection in women using HRT, but it actually appears to protect against the development of endometrial cancer in all postmenopausal women.

In the same study, women using no HRT at all were at higher risk than those on progesterone because of their own endogenous estrogen. These women developed 245.5 cases per 100,000 women per year. Not only has the rate of cancer declined with the use of progesterone, but those women who develop it tend to do so at a later age.

Reduces Hot Flashes. Progesterone used alone can relieve hot flashes and other vasomotor symptoms in about 60 to 80 percent of the women who use this therapy. Between 15 and 20 percent of women who are making the transition into menopause experience hot flashes even while they're still having fairly regular menstrual periods. Often these women also experience the heavy bleeding, premenstrual tension and other symptoms that characterize this stage.

Unfortunately, ERT cannot be used to suppress such hot flashes because many of these women have higher than normal levels of estrogen and, often, are not ovulating regularly. Thus, ERT used alone could intensify the pre-existing state of hormonal imbalance. Progesterone can also be used to relieve hot flashes in women who are clearly postmenopausal, but for varying reasons cannot use estrogen (such as estrogen allergy or large uterine fibroid tumors).

Prevents or Treats Osteoporosis. Although estrogen helps prevent osteoporosis by inhibiting calcium loss from the bone, the addition of progesterone helps decrease calcium loss even more effectively; it also promotes new bone formation. As a result, progesterone therapy actually increases bone mass.

A number of studies have suggested that natural progesterone may be effective in protecting women from osteoporosis. John R. Lee, M.D., has done much research into the use of progesterone to reverse osteoporosis. The results of one of his studies were published in the *International Clinical Nutrition Review*. Dr. Lee selected 100 Caucasian, postmenopausal women between the ages of 38 and 83. The average age was 65.2 at the beginning of the study. The majority of the women had already experienced some loss of height due to osteoporosis.

They were instructed to use conjugated estrogen (0.3 to 0.625 mg per day for three weeks each month) and progesterone (a 3 percent topical cream applied daily to the skin for 12 days each month or during the last two weeks of estrogen use). The women were also given a dietary and exercise program to follow, as well as vitamin and mineral supplements. Alcohol consumption was limited, and no smoking was allowed. The bone health of the women was followed for at least three years.

All the women in the study experienced some degree of progressive increase in bone mineral density, as well as improvement in such clinical symptoms as height stabilization, pain relief, and an increase in physical activity. During the course of the study, there were also no fractures due to osteoporosis. These improvements occurred independently of the women's ages.

The women commonly had an increase in the density of vertebral bone of 10 percent in the first six to 12 months of treatment. This increase was purportedly followed by additional yearly increases of 3 to 5 percent. This degree of bone remineralization over a relatively short period of time constitutes an exceptionally good therapeutic response.

Other Benefits of Natural Progesterone are equally beneficial. It functions as a diuretic and an anti-anxiety treatment. It can also stimulate libido, help prevent and treat fibrocystic breast disease, regulate thyroid hormone activity, stabilize blood sugar levels, and assist in normal blood clotting. Plus, natural progesterone is essential for the production of cortisone in the adrenal cortex, and helps convert fat to energy.

Side Effects of Natural Progesterone. When natural progesterone is taken in normally prescribed amounts, there are no known side effects. However, very high doses can cause drowsiness, due to its sedative effect on the brain, and huge doses of the hormone can be an anesthetic or cause a person to feel drunk. During the beginning stages of supplementing with progesterone, a woman may have symptoms of estrogen dominance. This happens because progesterone can increase the sensitivity of estrogen receptor sites. However, this sensitivity will disappear after a few weeks.

10

Supplementing With Testosterone

The third bioidentical hormone replacement option of the major sex hormones in my program is to supplement your nutrient regimen with natural, biochemically identical testosterone. Bioidentical testosterone is quite effective, if needed, for the "heavy lifting" that the use of actual hormone replacement therapy provides. Now that bioidentical estrogen and progesterone hormone replacement therapy has become more generally accepted, countless numbers of women have also begun to supplement with testosterone.

At about age 20, a woman produces peak levels of estrogen, progesterone, and testosterone, but by the time she reaches midlife and passes through menopause, production of these hormones is greatly diminished. To remedy this, estrogen and progesterone are routinely prescribed to restore a woman to youthful hormone status. However, testosterone, which was very much a part of her original hormonal makeup, is much less commonly added into the mix.

Among those women who do decide to take this hormone, the most common reasons are its ability to help prevent vaginal discomfort and soreness while increasing sex drive. In my practice, I've seen testosterone rapidly restore libido (though not for all women), which is an issue for many of my patients, as it affects the pleasurable aspects of intimate relationships. Testosterone is also prescribed for postmenopausal women who are troubled by abnormally low body weight, poor musculature, poor coordination, and osteoporosis.

Natural, Bioidentical Testosterone

Natural testosterone is produced by compounding pharmacies, which are able to formulate a wide range of dosages. These can be prepared as a cream or a gel (the two most popular forms), or as sublingual tablets or oral capsules.

Creams

Most women's compounding pharmacies suggest using creams containing 0.5 mg/g to 1 mg/g of testosterone. One-quarter teaspoon provides 1 g of cream and 0.5 mg of testosterone. A typical dose is ⅛ - ¼ teaspoon, used daily in the morning. The cream is applied to various sites, which are rotated, including the inner thigh, the back of the hand, the abdomen, and the arm. An advantage of testosterone cream is that, once absorbed through the skin, it immediately enters the general circulation and travels directly to target cells. Only later does the testosterone pass through the liver, which then begins to metabolize, or break down, the hormone.

Rachael's Story

When Rachael came to see me, her most distressing complaint was her lack of libido and difficulty enjoying sex with her husband. She had gone through menopause at age 49, and now, one year later, she complained that her sex drive had not only evaporated, but intercourse was painful because her vaginal tissues would tear a bit during penetration.

Besides a powerful libido-enhancing nutritional program of DHEA, PABA, arginine, and other important nutrients, Rachael began using bioidentical estrogen and progesterone, as well as testosterone creams to build up her tissues. Within no time, sex became much more pleasurable once again.

Gels

The gel is normally applied to vaginal tissue, from which the testosterone is absorbed into the bloodstream.

Sublingual Tablets

Sublingual tablets are well absorbed. Women usually begin with doses of 2-5 mg, but even a dose of only 0.5 mg may be sufficient. A reduced dose may be appropriate for a woman who is also taking estrogen, because estrogen activates testosterone receptor sites and strengthens its hormonal effect.

Oral Capsules

Capsules can be prepared with no preservatives, which some people prefer. However, capsules do have a disadvantage in that, once absorbed; the testosterone must first pass through the liver before entering the general circulation. Because the liver metabolizes the hormone, a smaller quantity of less active testosterone reaches target cells.

Injections

In a double-blind, placebo-controlled trial of 107 women with active rheumatoid arthritis, which was published in the *Annals of the Rheumatic Diseases*, weekly supplemental testosterone injections brought significant improvement in comfort and quality of life. Arthritis can be quite a crippling and disabling health issue in severe cases in women during the postmenopausal years.

Medical Research on the Benefits of Testosterone

As you can imagine, much research has been done on the use of supplemental testosterone. Unfortunately, most of this research has been performed using synthetic versions of the hormone. However, I and other like-minded alternative and complementary medicine physicians believe that biochemically identical testosterone has the same benefits found with the synthetic versions, but is a healthier hormonal option.

One study published in the *American Journal of Obstetrics and Gynecology* found that women who had received a total hysterectomy, including removal of their ovaries, benefited greatly from testosterone supplementation. As the ovaries make one-third of the testosterone in the female body, their removal causes a significant decline in testosterone production. The women were divided into four groups and given combined estrogen and androgen, one or the other of the hormones alone, or a placebo. The treatments were administered for three months, followed by a differing treatment for another three months. There was also a control group of ten women who underwent hysterectomy, but retained their ovaries. The women receiving androgen therapy, alone or with estrogen, and the women with ovarian function intact reported significantly higher ratings of energy and well-being than those women not receiving androgens.

Another study cited in a review article appearing in the *Journal of Clinical Endocrinology and Metabolism* found that testosterone cream or the oral estrogen/testosterone combination therapy can significantly increase sex drive. Women who had had their ovaries surgically removed were injected with testosterone enanthate (a synthetic) and reported an increase in the intensity of sexual arousal, sexual interest, and frequency of sexual fantasies above the effect they experienced taking only estrogen. Similarly, a study from the *Journal of Clinical Endocrinology and Metabolism* cited several controlled studies also documenting an increased intensity of sexual drive, sexual arousal, and frequency of sexual fantasies in women receiving testosterone supplementation.

Additionally, testosterone has a positive effect on a variety of psychological symptoms. In a study from the *American Journal of Obstetrics and Gynecology*, patients completed a daily questionnaire, rating such items as feeling blue and depressed, crying spells, needless worry, and loss of interest in life. Those women receiving testosterone reported negative feelings significantly less frequently than women not receiving the hormone.

Research from the journal *Menopause* confirms these findings. The study tested the effects of an SSRI (selective serotonin reuptake inhibitor) antidepressant versus a combination of various hormonal therapies. Researchers divided 72 postmenopausal, depressed women into four groups. One group received the antidepressant alone, another received the antidepressant with a synthetic estrogen/progesterone combination, the third took a synthetic testosterone with the antidepressant, and the fourth received a combination of all four drugs.

At the end of 24 weeks, only 48 women were still involved in the trial. Of the remaining women, researchers found that they all enjoyed relief from their menopausal symptoms. However, only those women who took the antidepressant with the testosterone reported an improvement in mood.

Testosterone supplementation can also improve your physical health, including menopausal symptoms and osteoporosis. A small study, reported in *American Family Physician* and presented at the sixth annual meeting of the North American Menopause Society, monitored two groups of women experiencing menopausal symptoms. One group of 12 women were each given 1.25 mg of estrogen daily, while a second group of 13 women were each given the same dosage of estrogen and 2.5 mg of methyltestosterone.

While both treatments had a positive effect on vaginal dryness and hot flashes, only the combined therapy helped relieve associated nervousness, irritability, fatigue, and insomnia. Other studies have shown that combined hormone therapy is also more effective in improving sleep quality and energy levels.

In another study from *Obstetrics and Gynecology*, 66 women who had undergone surgical menopause were given estrogen either alone or combined with testosterone. While both treatments prevented loss of bone in the spine and hip, only the combined therapy produced a significant increase in bone mineral density in the spine.

Side-Effects of Testosterone Therapy

The downside of supplementing with testosterone is that, when taken in high amounts, masculinization can occur. Your voice may deepen, you may develop more facial hair, and there may be clitoral enlargement. Acne may develop, and existing skin problems can worsen. You may also experience changes in your menstrual cycle, and if you are pregnant and take testosterone, a female fetus can develop male sexual characteristics. However, these effects are not likely to happen when testosterone is administered in the smaller, safer dosages appropriate for women.

There is also a possibility that testosterone may increase your risk of heart disease, and if taken with estrogen, testosterone may neutralize some of the benefits of estrogen therapy. Testosterone lowers "good" HDL cholesterol, a risk factor for cardiac problems. There is some evidence that testosterone given by injection, rather than given orally, is able to maintain more healthful levels of HDL.

It is important for anyone taking testosterone to be monitored closely by a physician so that any adverse effects can be recognized and dealt with promptly. Maintaining optimum testosterone levels not only improves your libido and enhances your mood; it also protects your heart and bones. By following the program I've outlined in this chapter, you can maintain proper testosterone balance for years to come.

11

General Guidelines of Bioidentical Hormone Replacement Therapy Use

In this chapter, I share with you guidelines that I have found to be of great benefit when prescribing these therapies to patients. I recommend that you understand and follow these principles if you wish to obtain the best results from HRT. These relate to dosage, route of administration, regimen and frequency, choice of physician, and proper cessation.

Choose the Lowest Dose that Works

In general, use the lowest possible dosage of both estrogen and progesterone that will relieve your symptoms and prevent long term health problems associated with hormonal deficiency such as osteoporosis and cardiovascular disease. If you start at higher doses, you are more likely to encounter side effects such as anxiety, mood swings, fluid retention and breast tenderness. Many women who could benefit from HRT discontinue it because of unpleasant (and often unnecessary) side effects.

Some women find that even the tiniest dosage of estrogen normally prescribed provides adequate symptom relief. However, such a low dosage may not provide sufficient protection against the development of bone loss or cardiovascular disease. Thus, women with high risk factors for developing either problem should not use this minimal dosage.

To know your risk potential, have your physician perform the appropriate tests. If you feel comfortable at the smaller dosages, you may wish to combine bioidentical estrogen with the alternative therapies described later in this book. At the other end of the spectrum, you may feel your best only when using estrogen in the high-dose ranges. If you have experienced a surgical menopause below the age of 40, you may need more estrogen than women who go through natural menopause at a later age. Obviously, with estrogen, one dosage does not fit all women and therapy must be carefully individualized to each woman's needs.

Progesterone should also be used in the lowest possible dose to prevent side effects. This is particularly true for the synthetic progestins, which can cause the most problems. Your physician will order the lowest dose to confer protection against uterine cancer, yet one that is comfortable for you. This may require some fine-tuning and tests such as a vaginal ultrasound under the guidance of your physician.

Choose the Route of Administration that Is Most Comfortable

Some women find it difficult to remember to take one or two pills each day. They may, occasionally, miss days. This does not create the same potential problem that missing a day or two of birth control pills will, because menopausal women do not have to worry about unplanned pregnancies (unless they are in the early stages of menopause). However, if you find pill-taking too challenging or unpleasant, then you are better off asking your physician about the alternative routes of administration such as the estrogen transdermal patch or progesterone cream.

Choose the HRT Regimen that Suits You Best

Traditionally, estrogen was taken only three weeks per month with one week off. Provera, a common progestin, was added during the last 10 to 13 days of the regimen to prevent the development of endometrial cancer. Taking one week off estrogen each month reduces the time during which the uterine lining is exposed to estrogen, therefore, reducing the risk.

However, some women find that menopausal symptoms, such as hot flashes, recur during this "off" week. In addition, many women dislike the bleeding, similar to a regular menstrual period, that occurs within a few days after the hormones are stopped. Even though the bleeding tends to be lighter and even diminishes or stops over time, many women find it an annoyance.

While some physicians still use the traditional three weeks on, one week off regimen with their patients, other regimens have become very popular in recent years. With one protocol, estrogen is taken every day and a progestin is added on an intermittent basis, usually during the first 12 days of the calendar month. More than two-thirds of the women on this regimen, if they have a uterus, experience bleeding when administration of progestin stops after the twelfth day. With combined continuous therapy, both estrogen and low doses of progestins are used on a daily basis without stopping. Women on this regimen may experience irregular bleeding during the first six months of treatment, which then diminishes.

With both continuous and combined continuous therapy regimens, bleeding often doesn't persist indefinitely. For many women, bleeding becomes lighter and stops entirely after a few years. This occurs as the endometrium eventually becomes inactive.

Both these regimens appear to protect women against the development of uterine cancer as well as does the "on-off regimen". Also, constant daily hormonal intake protects women better from recurrence of menopausal symptoms.

Pick a Physician Who Will Tailor HRT to Your Needs

One of the most important factors in developing a successful menopause relief program is to work with a physician who is knowledgeable and dedicated to helping you achieve the best therapeutic results. How does one find such a physician? You might try asking your friends for a referral. Choose several physicians and interview them to determine if their philosophy of HRT and personality fit with you. Ask many questions and evaluate the responses. Remember, this relationship between you and your physician will be a long-term one.

Attaining the goal of the best HRT regimen for you may require considerable tinkering over time with both dosages and formulations until the right results are achieved. Though some women adapt easily and effortlessly to their hormonal regimen, others need the expertise and help of an empathetic physician to achieve the results they desire. However, if you have made the decision to use HRT and believe strongly that these hormones can provide you with real benefits, it is worth the time and persistence. The benefits that HRT can provide are discussed in detail in the following chapters.

Stop Hormone Use Gradually

What if you've been on HRT for some time and now feel that it's time to stop using it? While many women stay on HRT indefinitely, other women do not feel the need to continue with HRT after using it for a short period of time. Once the initial symptoms are relieved and the body is adjusted to the postmenopausal period, they may wish to see how they feel without hormones. Others dislike the side effects that develop with HRT, so choose to discontinue it. Whatever the reason for stopping HRT, don't do it abruptly. This can cause a severe recurrence of symptoms (such as hot flashes) as your body reacts to the rapid decline in estrogen. Just as during the early postmenopausal period, the pituitary pumps out high levels of FSH in an attempt to make your body produce the estrogen that has suddenly disappeared. Hot flashes and night sweats can reappear as the pituitary-hypothalamic axis goes off balance.

Be sure to stop HRT use very slowly. I often recommend cutting the dose of estrogen by one-half each month for one or two months. Then cut back to every other day for a month, followed by twice a week for a month, and finally to once a week for a month. Continue to take your progesterone on your regular schedule until you have stopped the estrogen entirely, then discontinue it. If your symptoms recur in too uncomfortable a fashion, you can always begin HRT use again.

Using HRT in the safest and most comfortable dosage and regimen for your individual needs will provide the best therapeutic results with the least risks and side effects. What you can expect in terms of symptom relief from your HRT program is discussed in the next chapter.

Part III:
Alternatives to Hormone Replacement Therapy

12

Dietary Principles for Menopause Relief

Diet plays a very important role in determining the health of menopausal women. The foods you choose may trigger hot flashes and other unpleasant menopausal symptoms, as well as increase your risk of developing such serious diseases as heart attacks, strokes, cancer and arthritis. On the other hand, foods chosen wisely for their high nutrient content and easy digestibility can decrease and even prevent symptoms of menopause.

The traditional American diet tends to work against us, because it is laden with unhealthy fat, sugar, salt and stimulants. If you follow this diet without making modifications as your body ages, your health will suffer. To change your eating habits in ways that will help create optimal health and well-being during your menopausal years requires knowledge about important concepts of nutrition, much of which never gets applied to the lives of many women in menopause.

This chapter contains essential information about diet that you may use to change your own habits toward optimal health. I have used these guidelines with my patients and they have been delighted with the beneficial results. The first section discusses the foods that you should emphasize for good health. In the second section, I will provide information on which foods to avoid or limit.

Foods That Ease Menopausal Symptoms

This diet emphasizes high-nutrient foods such as beans and peas (legumes), whole grains, foods containing essential and healthy fatty acid-containing foods (including raw seeds and nuts), certain fish, poultry, eggs, and lots of fresh fruits and vegetables. There is evidence that this dietary approach can help relieve and prevent symptoms of menopause. These types of foods predominate in the traditional diets of many Asian and African cultures. Interestingly, menopausal symptoms tend to be much less prevalent and severe in these cultures. For example, these symptoms occur in 10 to 15 percent of Japanese women at midlife, in contrast with 80 to 85 percent of American women. Diet is thought to play a major role in the different ways women experience menopausal symptoms. Let us look at the benefits each of the healthy foods can bring you during your midlife years.

Beans and Peas (Legumes)

Soybean-based products actually help reduce and prevent menopausal symptoms. Soybeans are loaded with natural plant or phytoestrogens, called isoflavones. The estrogen-like isoflavones, particularly genistein and daidzein, were identified decades ago by researchers. Large quantities of soybeans are consumed in the traditional Japanese diet, providing as much as 30 to 100 mg of isoflavones per day. This may be one reason that the women report fewer menopausal problems.

As weak estrogens, these compounds bind to estrogen receptors and act as a substitute form of estrogen in the body. Although menopausal women are deficient in estrogen, the isoflavones can help reduce common symptoms, such as hot flashes and vaginal dryness. In addition, isoflavone-containing foods may also have an anticarcinogenic effect, which could explain the lower incidence of breast cancer among Japanese women and lower mortality from prostate cancer among Japanese men.

U.S. studies have confirmed the benefits of a soy-rich diet in reducing the risk of breast cancer. For example, a study reported in the *American Journal of Epidemiology* found that women who had the highest consumption of legumes were fifty-four percent less likely to develop uterine cancer.

Dietary studies show that men, women and children in Japan, as well as Americans following a macrobiotic diet or vegetarian diet, excrete 100 to 1000 times more isoflavones in their urine than people in Finland and the United States who eat a meat and dairy-based diet, which has an isoflavone content eighty percent lower than a vegetarian-based diet.

A study published in the *British Medical Journal* described how shifting the diet towards phytoestrogen-containing foods can change certain menopause indicators. In this study, twenty-five menopausal women (average age of fifty-nine) supplemented their normal diet with phytoestrogen-containing foods such as soy flour, flaxseed oil and red clover sprouts over a six-week period. Smears from the vaginal wall were taken every two weeks to see if the addition of estrogen-containing plant foods would cause a beneficial hormonal effect on the vagina. Typically, the vaginal mucosa thins out and becomes more prone to trauma and infections with menopause. Interestingly, the vaginal mucosa responded positively to the ingestion of soy flour and flax oil, but returned to previous levels eight weeks after these foods were discontinued.

Another study involved eighty postmenopausal women who are were given either soy (with premeasured phytoestrogen content) or Premarin (the most frequently prescribed form of estrogen in the United States). Both the soy and estrogen were found to have beneficial effects on both blood fats and bone metabolism. Soy isoflavones are currently available in capsule or powder forms as nutritional supplements. Optimally, a woman should ingest from 30 to 60 mg per day.

Legumes in general are excellent foods for menopausal women. Common sources include garbanzo beans, kidney beans, lima beans, black beans and lentils. All legumes are an excellent source of protein. When combined with whole grains, the two foods provide the full range of essential amino acids, the building blocks of protein.

In addition, legumes are an excellent source of fiber. This enables their nutrients, such as protein and carbohydrates, to be absorbed more slowly. This has many health benefits. The slow digestion of legume-based carbohydrates can help regulate the blood sugar level. As a result, legumes are an excellent food for women with blood sugar imbalances or diabetes. The fiber can help normalize bowel function and lower cholesterol levels by promoting excretion of cholesterol through the bowel movements.

Legumes are excellent sources of many other nutrients needed by menopausal women. These include calcium and magnesium, which are essential for strong bones and healthy muscle tone. Legumes also contain high levels of potassium, which help regulate the heartbeat as well as provide muscle tone. Legumes are very high in iron, copper and zinc. Sufficient iron intake is particularly important for women with heavy menstrual bleeding who are beginning menopause. Legumes are also high in vitamin B-complex, essential for healthy liver function. The liver metabolizes estrogen so that it can be excreted efficiently from the body.

Whole Grains

Healthy grains for menopausal women include oats, corn, barley, millet, quinoa, buckwheat, wild rice, brown rice and whole wheat. As with legumes, many whole grains are an excellent source of phytoestrogens. Whole grains contain lignans, a material that is used to form the plant cell wall. Lignans, like isoflavones, are weakly estrogenic and can provide additional nutritional support to menopausal women deficient in this hormone.

In addition, certain grain-like plants such as buckwheat are good sources of another flavonoid called rutin. This flavonoid is particularly helpful in its ability to strengthen capillaries and reduce heavy menstrual bleeding when women are just entering menopause. Flavonoids, like rutin, along with vitamin C, have been used in medical studies to reduce heavy bleeding during this time, and for bleeding due to fibroid tumors and spontaneous abortions. One study of women who miscarried multiple pregnancies concluded that the bioflavonoid-vitamin C combination allowed seventy-eight percent of high-risk women studied to carry their pregnancies to full term.

The high fiber content of whole grains also helps regulate estrogen levels because of the ability of fiber to bind estrogen in the intestinal tract and remove it from the body through bowel movements. As described earlier, estrogen circulates in the blood throughout the body, including the liver. The liver metabolizes estrogen from its more potent forms, estradiol and estrone, to a chemically inactive and weaker form, estriol. When the liver is functioning in a healthy manner, this occurs efficiently. The estrogen metabolites are then secreted into the bile and from there into the digestive tract. This whole process is called the enterohepatic circulation of estrogen.

A high-fat, low-fiber diet promotes the growth of certain bacteria in the intestinal tract that act chemically on these estrogen products. These bacteria convert the estrogen products back to estrone and estradiol, allowing reabsorption of the estrogen back into the body. As mentioned earlier in this book, estrone is the primary type of estrogen produced by the body after menopause, and estradiol is the type of estrogen produced by the ovary during the active reproductive years.

As a result of the intestinal bacteria, the levels of these two estrogens rise higher than estriol, their primary breakdown product. This abundance of the more potent forms of estrogen may not present a healthy estrogen profile. Research studies have shown that estradiol and estrone, as the more chemically active and potent forms of estrogen, may predispose women toward developing breast cancer, while estriol, a much weaker form of estrogen, may confer protection against breast cancer. Thus, a high-fiber, low-fat diet may help regulate not only the estrogen levels, but the types of estrogen circulating through a woman's body. A number of studies have shown that vegetarian women excrete two to three times more estrogen in their bowel movements than do women eating the typical high-fat, low-fiber diet.

Besides regulating estrogen levels, the high-fiber content of whole grains binds to cholesterol, increasing its excretion from the body through the digestive tract. This helps lower blood cholesterol levels, reducing a significant risk factor for heart attacks in postmenopausal women. The fiber in grain is very helpful in relieving constipation, as well as preventing other diseases of the digestive tract such as diverticulitis and hiatus hernia. Fiber may also have a protective effect against developing colon cancer, a disease also found more commonly in people who eat a high-fat, low-fiber diet.

Whole grains are excellent sources of carbohydrates capable of stabilizing blood sugar and helping eliminate sugar craving. They help prevent or control diabetes mellitus, a dangerous disease that predisposes people toward heart disease, blood vessel problems, infections and blindness. Fifty percent of our population over age 60 have blood sugar abnormalities, due in great part to the tremendous amount of high-sugared foods and sweets Americans eat. Whole grains, with their natural sweetness, can satisfy much of this craving in a healthful way.

In addition, whole grains are a major source of complete protein when combined in a meal with legumes. Whole grains also contain many excellent nutrients for menopausal women. They contain high levels of vitamin B and vitamin E, both of which are critical for healthy hormonal balance and regulating estrogen levels. This occurs through their beneficial effect on both the liver and ovaries. Whole grains' vitamin B and vitamin E content also help combat the fatigue and depression that can occur with the onset of menopause. Grains are high in magnesium, which helps reduce muscle tension. They are also high in calcium, necessary for healthy bones and to relax muscle tension. Finally, whole grains are high in potassium. Potassium has a diuretic effect on body tissues and helps reduce bloating, which can be a problem for postmenopausal women.

Essential Fatty Acid-Containing Foods

Healthy essential oils are extremely beneficial for menopausal women. Linoleic acid, a member of the omega-6 family of fatty acids, is primarily found in raw seeds and nuts. Good sources include flaxseed, pumpkin seeds, sesame seeds, sunflower seeds and walnuts. EPA (eicosapentaenoic acid) and DHA (docosahexaenoic acid) are members of the omega-3 family and are primarily found in certain fish such as trout, salmon, mackerel. Alpha-linolenic acid is a member of the omega-3 family as well and found in some plant sources like flaxseeds, soy, pumpkin seeds, walnuts and green leafy vegetables. Both essential fatty acid families must be derived from dietary sources because they cannot be produced by the body.

The body does not primarily burn the essential fatty acids for energy, unlike the saturated fats found in red meat, eggs, dairy products, and a few plants such as palm oil. Instead, these fatty acids have special functions in the body necessary for good health and survival. The skin is full of fatty acids that, along with estrogen, provide moisture, softness and smooth texture. When the estrogen levels decline with menopause, moisture can continue to be provided to the skin, vagina and bladder mucosa by increasing levels of fatty acid-containing foods. Flaxseed oil is particularly good for dry skin because it contains high levels of both fatty acids. In addition, fatty acids are a main structural component of all cell membranes and are found in high levels in such important tissues as the brain and nerve cells, retina of the eye, adrenal gland and inner ear.

Besides relieving tissue dryness, essential fatty acids are also needed by the body as precursors for the production of important hormone-like chemicals called prostaglandins. There are over 30 types of prostaglandins manufactured by tissues throughout the body. The proper balance of prostaglandins can play a major role in relieving and preventing many diseases that occur predominantly in the postmenopausal period.

The series one prostaglandins are manufactured by the body from linoleic acid. These prostaglandins have many beneficial effects. One member of the series, called prostaglandin E, or PGE, is particularly helpful for menopausal women. It relaxes the blood vessels and improves circulation. It keeps the platelets, a component of blood, from sticking or clumping together. This reduces the likelihood of heart attacks and strokes by preventing blood clotting and obstruction of the blood vessels. Since the incidence of heart attacks increases ten-fold between the ages of 55 and 65, PGE can benefit women greatly. In addition, PGE prevents inflammation, reducing the symptoms of arthritis. For many women, arthritis symptoms begin after they go through menopause. PGE also stimulates the immune system and helps insulin function effectively.

The series-3 prostaglandins are manufactured from the eicosapentaenoic acid (EPA) found in fish such as salmon and trout. They are also produced more slowly from plant sources containing alpha-linolenic acid. As mentioned earlier, flax oil is a particularly good food source of alpha-linolenic acid. One member of this series called PGE 3 has anticlotting effects similar to those of PGE. They also help reduce the likelihood of heart attacks and strokes when manufactured by the body in high levels. PGE 3 also decreases triglycerides levels, another risk factor for heart attacks.

It also helps prevent the manufacture of PGE 2, an undesirable prostaglandin made from arachidonic acid, a fatty acid derived primarily from dietary sources of red meat and dairy products. Unlike PGE and PGE 3, arachidonic acid-derived PGE 2 actually promotes platelet aggregation or clumping, thereby initiating potentially dangerous clot formation. It also causes inflammation and fluid retention, which can predispose postmenopausal women towards arthritis and high blood pressure.

In addition, the use of trans fatty acid containing foods like margarine have been shown to increase C-reactive protein, an important marker of inflammation and heart disease, in a study of more than 700 nurses. These types of foods should be avoided. Thus, it is important to favor fish, seeds and nuts as sources of protein to promote production of the "good" prostaglandins.

Fish, Poultry and Eggs

Fish, poultry and eggs are the best choices for women who feel their best and have more energy and vitality eating a meat based diet. A number of people simply enjoy the flavor and texture of meat, while some of my patients have told me that they actually don't feel as well or as energized on an all-vegetarian diet.

If you fall into one of these categories, fish, poultry and eggs can supply a number of important nutritional needs. They are excellent sources of high-quality protein. All types of fish, including saltwater fish, freshwater fish, and shellfish, as well as all types of commonly eaten poultry like chicken, turkey, duck, goose, and game fowl, as well as eggs contain a complete range of the essential amino acids needed to build protein. These acids can be utilized by the body for many purposes, such as building structural components of tissue and maintaining immune function.

Many fish are also excellent sources of polyunsaturated fats, which provide tremendous health benefits. The best fish sources of these fats include salmon, trout, mackerel, and halibut.

Fish oils, including eicosapentaenoic acid (EPA) and docosahexaenoic acid (DHA), are converted to the series-3 prostaglandin hormones. One member of the series, called PGE 3, has anticlotting effects and helps to reduce platelet stickiness. As a result, it helps reduce the likelihood of heart attacks and strokes when it is manufactured by the body in high levels. PGE 3 also helps to decrease triglyceride levels, thereby reducing another risk factor for heart attacks. It also helps prevent the manufacture of PGE 2, an undesirable prostaglandin made from arachidonic acid, which is a fatty acid derived primarily from dietary sources of red meat and dairy products. Unlike PGE 3, arachidonic acid-derived PGE 2 actually promotes platelet aggregation or clumping, thereby initiating potentially dangerous clot formation.

Series 3 prostaglandins are also important for the prevention and treatment of many common women's health issues. They needed for healthy ovulation and the production of progesterone during the second half of the menstrual cycle. As a result, they help to prevent estrogen dominant related health issues like fibroid tumors of the uterus, endometriosis, ovarian cysts, benign breast disease, PMS and heavy and irregular menstrual bleeding. These conditions are very common during the premenopause transition. Research studies have also found fish oil to be very helpful in reducing menstrual cramps and pain.

The major drawback with eating large amounts of fish is the high level of mercury found in a number of fish. Mercury is an extremely dangerous contaminant and can cause neurological damage, impair memory and cognitive function, cause chronic fatigue, and damage the heart, liver, and immune system. It is a very toxic heavy metal that accumulates in larger fish like tuna, shark, swordfish, pickerel, certain bass and other fish. As a result, I recommend eating fish no more than once or twice and week despite their many health benefits and supplementing instead on a daily basis with fish oil capsules. I recommend a total of 2000-3000 mg per day of the healthful omega-3 fatty acids, EPA and DHA, taken in fish oil capsules. It is very important to check the label of the fish oil supplements that you use to confirm the actual dosage of omega-3 fatty acids EPA and DHA that the product contains. Often, the amount of EPA and DHA contained in the product is much less than the total amount of the fish oil. It is important to check labels, of course, when taking any nutritional supplement to make sure that the dosages are at therapeutic levels.

Fish oil may need to be avoided in people on blood thinners like Coumadin, which is used medically for treating blood clots and strokes. This is because fish oil also has a blood thinning effect within the body. While this can be beneficial for normal people, it may be dangerous for these patients.

The fats found in poultry are a different story. While poultry such as turkey, chicken, and goose do contain some of the beneficial linoleic acid, the amount is much less than that found in plant sources. Linoleic acid ranges between 15 to 20 percent of the total fat content of turkey and chicken and 20 to 25 percent in goose. Certain fish (like salmon and trout) are far better sources of essential fatty acids than poultry. Luckily, much of poultry's fat is found within the skin (which is laden with fat) and in the internal organs, so it can be easily removed. In addition, the total fat content of the most commonly eaten poultry—chicken, and turkey—is far lower than that of beef (11 percent for chicken, compared to 30 to 40 percent for beef).

If you want to minimize your fat intake when eating poultry, choose muscle meat like breast and thigh over the internal organs, and remove the skin before cooking or eating. Also, it is best to eat white meat rather than dark, as white meat is much lower in fat. Also, avoid duck and goose, which tend to contain more fat in their meat and skins.

Besides protein and fat, fish and poultry contain a number of other important nutrients. Fatty fish, such as salmon and halibut, are good sources of vitamins A and D. Mackerel, herring, and haddock tend to be rich in minerals, although this varies by type of fish. Saltwater fish and shellfish are excellent sources of iodine, a difficult-to-obtain trace mineral needed for healthy thyroid function. They are also high in zinc—particularly oysters, though lobster and crab are fairly abundant in zinc as well. Shellfish are also a good source of selenium and copper. In general, fish provide high quantities of potassium, phosphorus, and iron, though magnesium levels tend to be low. Fish can be an excellent source of calcium. Canned sardines and salmon are good choices because of their tiny, partially dissolved and easily digested bones.

Chicken and turkey are less abundant in their vitamin and mineral content, for the most part, than fish or vegetable sources. Chicken does contain some vitamin A and vitamin B complex, but no vitamin E and negligible amounts of vitamin C. It does contain some potassium, phosphorus, sodium, zinc, and iron, but levels of other minerals like calcium, magnesium, and manganese tend to be low.

Turkey is fairly similar to chicken in its nutrient make up. A few minerals, such as potassium and phosphorus, are slightly more abundant in turkey than in chicken, but turkey's vitamin A content is even lower. Neither type of poultry should be used to supply all of your vitamin and mineral needs. They should be combined with plant-based foods such as fruits, vegetables, and whole grains, which are richer in these essential micronutrients. The same is true, to a lesser extent, with seafood.

Eggs are among my favorite food. While eggs from many different sources are available including duck, quail, and ostrich eggs, most people in our society prefer eating chicken eggs. Eggs are an excellent source of protein and are low in calories, containing only 70 to 80 calories each. Eggs also contain essential nutrients like iron, choline, vitamins A, B12, D and E as well as lutein and zeaxanthin, which are important for healthy vision.

While the egg yolk does contain saturated fat, even eating one egg a day does not appear to increase your risk of heart disease. This is according to the landmark study on nurses done through the Harvard University School of Public Health. Eggs also tend to be very filling because of their protein and fat content and can satisfy overweight individuals who are on weight loss program.

I recommend buying eggs from chickens that are raised free-range or cage free. Lower cholesterol eggs are also available from chickens fed a vegetarian diet and eggs that are rich in omega 3 fatty acids are being produced form chickens that are fed flaxseed, fish oil, and marine algae. These types of eggs are readily available from health food stores and some supermarkets.

Seafood and poultry can be purchased fresh, frozen, canned, and smoked. Seafood is also available cured and dried. Both seafood and poultry are prone to bacterial contamination and can cause infections to the consumer if not handled properly. Neither type of meat should be left out at room temperature. They should be well wrapped, refrigerated, and eaten soon after purchasing or thawing.

Both fish and poultry are best eaten broiled, roasted, sautéed, or baked. Frying or sautéing in large amounts of fat should be avoided. Poultry is rarely eaten raw, although seafood in sushi bars and in some seafood recipes calls for it to be served raw or only lightly cooked. There is some risk of contamination by parasites and bacteria when eating raw or undercooked seafood. It is important that any seafood eaten this way be as fresh and clean as possible.

If you eat poultry frequently, try to buy the organic, free range brands, as their exposure to pesticides, antibiotics, and hormones has been reduced. Also, I recommend limiting your intake of meat to moderate portions (6 - 8 ounces or less per day).

Most Americans eat much more protein than is healthy. Excessive amounts of protein are difficult to digest and stress the kidneys. Instead of using meat as your only source of protein, increase your intake of grains, beans, raw seeds, and nuts, which contain not only protein but also many other important nutrients. For many years I have recommended that my patients use meat more as a garnish and a flavoring for stir-fries and soups.

Vegetables

Vegetables are excellent foods that come in a wide variety of flavors, colors and textures. They are important for health because they are extremely rich in many vitamins and minerals. Recent research in the past two decades has also emphasized their importance in protecting postmenopausal women from diseases such as heart attacks, strokes, cancer and immune system breakdown.

Vegetables high in vitamin A usually have an orange, red or dark green color. These include squash, sweet potatoes, pepper, carrots, kale and lettuce, as well as many other common foods. Unlike animal-based sources of vitamin A, which contain an oil-soluble form of this vitamin, plant sources contain a precursor form of vitamin A called beta-carotene. Beta-carotene is converted to vitamin A by the liver and intestines once ingested into the body. This form tends to be very safe and is found in high doses in many foods. For example, one glass of carrot juice or a sweet potato each contains 20,000 international units [IU] of beta-carotene. Many people eat two to three times this amount in their daily diet.

Research shows that vitamin A will protect against cancer and immune system deficiency. Of particular interest to menopausal women are studies showing that vitamin A may protect against breast cancer. Other research studies suggest that a high intake of plant foods containing beta-carotene protects against heart attacks in high-risk people.

Many vegetables are also high in vitamin C, which has a protective effect against heart attack, cancer, and immune system problems. Vitamin C is particularly important for transitional menopausal women because, along with iron and bioflavonoids, it can protect against excessive menopausal bleeding. Research studies also suggest that vitamin C may help protect women from developing cervical cancer as well as vitamin A does. Vitamin C is important for wound healing and healthy skin. Vegetables high in vitamin C include potatoes, pepper, peas, tomatoes, broccoli, brussels sprouts, cabbage, cauliflower, kale and parsley.

Vegetables contain many other important nutrients such as iron, magnesium and calcium that protect against osteoporosis, anemia and excessive menstrual bleeding. Leafy green vegetables, such as beet greens, collards and dandelion greens, are excellent sources of these important nutrients. Other vegetables also have health enhancing properties. Onions and garlic decrease the blood's clotting tendency and lower serum cholesterol, which can help decrease the incidence of stroke and heart attack. Studies indicate that ginger root, onions and mushrooms may have a similar effect.

Certain mushrooms may even stimulate immune system function. Some vegetables such as kelp are high in iodine and trace minerals, essential for healthy thyroid function. Use kelp as a seasoning to sprinkle on vegetables and grains. Finally, vegetable fiber contributes to healthy bowl function and regulates levels of cholesterol and estrogen. It also promotes more efficient excretion of fat and estrogen through the intestinal tract. Be sure to eat your vegetables raw or lightly steamed to preserve their nutrient value. Do not boil or overcook vegetables, because vitamins and minerals can be lost through improper preparation.

Fruits

Fruits are an exceptional source of bioflavonoids and vitamin C, which helps to control excessive menstrual flow as well as provide the body with weak plant sources of estrogen. The inner peel and pulp of the citrus fruit is an excellent source of bioflavonoids and, in fact, is used for commercial production of bioflavonoid supplements. This is, unfortunately, the more bitter part of the fruit that many women discard, unaware of the health benefits the inner peel and pulp can provide. Also, the skin of grapes, cherries and many berries are rich sources of bioflavonoids. So, it is better to eat the whole fruit rather than just drink the juice.

Adequate potassium intake is necessary for good health, and fruits are very good food sources of potassium. Potassium helps lower high blood pressure and protects against heart disease; it also decreases bloating and fluid retention. Medical studies show that potassium is beneficial in reducing menopause-related fatigue. Fruits high in potassium include bananas, oranges, grapefruits, berries, peaches, apricots and melons. Fruits are also an excellent source of vitamin C, which provides important protection against cancer and infectious diseases as well as heart disease. Most whole fruits contain some vitamin C—berries, oranges, and melons provide exceptionally high levels of this essential nutrient. Yellow and orange colored fruits such as papaya, persimmon, apricot and tangerine should be included in your diet because of their high vitamin C content.

Although fruit is high in sugar, the high fiber content of the whole fruit slows down digestion, curbs appetite and stabilizes the blood sugar level. The high fiber content of many fruits makes them excellent foods for women who experience constipation. A recent study published in the *Journal of the National Cancer Institute*, also found that a high intake of fruits and vegetables appears to confer some protection against developing breast cancer. This is because fiber seems to reduce levels of circulating estrogens by binding to estrogens in the intestines and promoting their excretion from the body through the bowel movements. Pineapple and papaya also contain enzymes that help to break down protein, so they promote good digestive function and speed up bowel transit time.

Be aware that fruit juice does not contain the bulk or fiber of whole fruit, so it does not stabilize blood sugar or have beneficial effects on bowel function. Juice acts more like the simple sugars found in candy, so it should be used sparingly. The whole fruit retains the sweet flavor and makes a healthy substitute for candies, cookies, cakes and other highly sugared foods. Use it as a snack or dessert instead of cookies, candies, pastries or ice cream.

Foods to Avoid or Limit with Menopause

Diet can have a negative effect on your health as you go through and beyond menopause, if your food selection is poorly chosen. Foods described in this section either accentuate menopausal symptoms or add to the risk of developing diseases that increase in incidence during the postmenopausal period. These include heart disease, stroke, high blood pressure, cancer, arthritis and diabetes, to name only the most common ones.

Caffeine-Containing Foods

Caffeine-containing foods include beverages such as coffee, black tea, cola drinks and chocolate. These foods are used almost universally in our culture, both as stimulants and as emotional "treats." Caffeine belongs to a class of chemicals called methylxanthines, central nervous stimulants that increase alertness and energy level. Many menopausal women use a caffeinated beverage on a regular basis to combat fatigue and provide a pick-up in the morning. This practice may accelerate during menopause when fatigue is often worse due to poor sleep quality. Hot flashes and perspiration can recur throughout the night, leaving women depleted of energy and exhausted.

Unfortunately, there are many negatives to the use of caffeinated beverages. Caffeine is an addictive chemical and a person often requires large amounts to provide wakefulness and alertness. Regular caffeine users who stop caffeine intake abruptly may experience withdrawal symptoms such as headaches, mood changes, and increased fatigue. Psychological symptoms such as anxiety, irritability and mood swings due to hormonal deficiency are increased with caffeine intake.

In addition, caffeine has a diuretic effect and increases the loss of many essential minerals and vitamins such as potassium, zinc, magnesium, vitamin B and vitamin C accelerates with caffeine intake. Coffee also reduces the absorption of iron and calcium from food and supplemental sources, particularly when used at mealtimes.

Several studies have confirmed caffeine as a significant contributor to osteoporosis. Discussed in a review article in the *Family Practice News*, this research found that consumption of more than three cups of coffee per day tripled the risk of hip fractures in susceptible women and also increased the risk of spinal fractures. Finally, caffeine use is linked to an increased incidence of nodules and tenderness in women with benign breast disease.

Postmenopausal women at high risk for a heart attack or stroke because of family tendency or blood fat profile may want to avoid caffeine. Caffeine increases blood cholesterol and triglyceride levels, risk factors for heart attacks. In addition, caffeine raises the blood pressure, another risk factor for heart attacks and strokes (hypertension becomes increasingly prevalent with age). Caffeine also causes the heart to beat faster and increases the excitability of the system that conducts electrical impulses through the heart. This can lead to irregular heartbeat in susceptible women.

Luckily, many substitutes are available for women who like either the taste of coffee or the pick-me-up that it produces. Water processed decaffeinated coffee is often the easiest substitute to start with for women who like the flavor of coffee. Coffee substitutes that are grain-based, such as Postum and Cafix, are even better and ginger tea can have a vitalizing and energetic effect.

Alcohol

Alcohol will intensify almost every type of menopausal symptom. As a result, I recommend that women with active symptoms limit their intake or avoid alcoholic beverages entirely. The list of symptoms of menopause affected by alcohol intake includes hot flashes and mood swings. Unlike caffeine, alcohol is a central nervous system depressant, so its intake can increase menopausal fatigue and depression. This is particularly pronounced in women with night sweats and insomnia whose sleep quality is already poor.

In addition, alcohol has a diuretic effect on the body. During our active reproductive years, estrogen helps keep the skin and other tissues plump by causing fluid and salt retention in the body. As our estrogen levels begin to wane, excessive intake of alcohol can further dehydrate the skin and tissues, including the vaginal and bladder mucosa. Alcohol's diuretic effect also causes the loss of excessive amounts of essential minerals through the urinary tract. These include minerals needed for healthy bones such as calcium, magnesium and zinc. Alcohol is also a contributor to osteoporosis. An article in the *Family Practice News* reviewed several studies on osteoporosis, which found that women who consumed more than seven ounces of alcohol per week nearly tripled their risk of hip fracture.

Alcohol irritates the liver. It is metabolized by the liver to a chemical called acetaldehyde, which is liver toxic. In addition, excessive alcohol cannot be metabolized to glucose or glycogen (the storage form of glucose). Instead, it is metabolized and stored in the liver as fat. Excessive fat deposition in the liver can eventually lead to scarring and cirrhosis. Excessive alcohol intake can also affect the liver's ability to metabolize estrogen and can elevate the body's blood estrogen levels, particularly of the more chemically active forms of estrogen.

On the positive side, alcohol in small amounts can be a pleasurable social beverage. When used in amounts not exceeding four ounces of wine, ten ounces of beer, or one ounce of hard liquor per day, it can have a pleasant, relaxing effect. It makes us more sociable and enhances the taste of food. Small amounts of alcohol may also increase the high-density lipoproteins, a type of blood fat that protects people against heart attacks. However, for optimal health, I recommend using alcohol no more than once or twice a week; this is true for women in midlife with no obvious menopausal symptoms.

Sugar

Sugar is one of the most overused foods in the United States. It is primarily utilized as a sweetening agent in the form of sucrose, which most of us know as white, granular table sugar. Sugar is a main ingredient of cookies, cakes, soft drinks, candies, ice cream, cereals and many other foods. Many women are unaware of how prevalent it is in convenience foods such as salad dressings, catsup, relish, and even some prepackaged main courses in the supermarket. Foods sold in natural food stores are highly sugared, too, although with different types of sweeteners such as fructose, maple syrup and honey. As a result of this national sweet tooth, the average American eats more than 120 pounds of sugar per year.

This dietary sugar is eventually metabolized to its simplest form in the body called glucose. Glucose by itself is essential for all cellular processes, because it is the major source of fuel our cells use to generate energy. However, when the body is flooded with too much sugar, it becomes overwhelmed, cannot process the sugar effectively and overreacts by pumping out large amounts of insulin. This is the hormone that helps drive glucose into the cells where it can be used as energy. When too much insulin is secreted, the blood sugar level falls, and hypoglycemia can occur. With continued overuse of sugar, the pancreas eventually "wears out" and is no longer able to clear sugar from the blood circulation efficiently. The blood sugar level rises and diabetes mellitus is the result. This tendency toward diabetes or high blood sugar levels increases dramatically after menopause. Research studies show that more than 50 percent of Americans have blood sugar imbalances by age 65.

Excess sugar intake also depletes the body's reserve of B-complex vitamins and many essential minerals by increasing their rate of utilization and sugar metabolism. This can increase anxiety, irritability and nervous tension that many women feel as they move into menopause. One research study even suggests that a diet high in sugar may impair liver function and affect the liver's ability to metabolize estrogen. Highly sugared foods also promote tooth decay and gum disease. Many women, however, are addicted to sugar and have a difficult time controlling their intake once they start eating sugary foods.

Because sugar is so deleterious to good health, menopausal women might consider avoiding sugar entirely or limiting its use to small amounts on social occasions. Sugar can be easily substituted in recipes by using fruit, sugar substitutes like stevia or brown rice syrup. Also, become a label reader. If canned and bottled foods such as salad dressings, soft drinks or baked beans have sugar near the top of the list, the product probably contains too much sugar. Search out alternatives that don't contain sugar or items using it in very small amounts. If you crave sweets, keep fresh or dried fruits handy such as apples, bananas or dried figs. Whole fruit should satisfy your craving for sweets and has the added benefit of being high in many essential nutrients.

Salt

Condiments and food additives such as table salt and monosodium glutamate (MSG) generally contain large amounts of sodium. Sodium is one of the body's major minerals. Primarily found in the body's extracellular compartment in conjunction with potassium, the primary intracellular mineral, sodium helps regulate water balance in the cells. Water tends to accumulate where sodium is prevalent. Thus, an overabundance of sodium relative to the body's potassium levels can lead to edema, bloating and sometimes high blood pressure. These problems are very common in menopausal women who are increasingly at risk for developing cardiovascular problems with age. In addition, fluid retention often adds to excess pounds that can be so irksome to women after menopause. Many women complain that they gain 10 to 15 pounds after menopause and that the weight is very difficult to lose, even with dieting and exercise. Of even greater concern is the fact that excess sodium is a risk factor for osteoporosis because it accelerates calcium loss from the body.

Unfortunately, as with sugar, salt is prevalent in the American diet. In fact, salt and sugar are often found together in large amounts in frozen and canned foods, cheeses, potato chips, hamburgers, hot dogs, cured meats, pizzas and other common foods. Many of us eat so much salt (far beyond the recommended 2000 mg or 1 teaspoon per day) that our palates have become jaded. Many people feel that food tastes too bland without the addition of salt.

Luckily, many other available seasoning options are much better for your health. For flavoring, use garlic, basil, oregano and other herbs. Fresh foods such as vegetables, grains, legumes and meat contain all the salt we need, so added table salt isn't necessary. As for sugar, read the labels before you buy bottled, canned or frozen food. Don't buy a product if salt is listed as a main ingredient (near the top of the list). Many brands in the health food stores and supermarkets now distribute foods labeled "no salt added" or "reduced salt content." Be sure to buy these rather than the high-salt content foods. Also, eat plenty of fresh fruits and vegetables because they are excellent sources of potassium and other essential nutrients. Potassium helps balance the sodium in the body and regulates the blood pressure to keep it at normal levels.

Red Meat, Dairy Products and Saturated Oils

At first glance, it may not be apparent that red meat, dairy products and saturated oils have much in common. However, they are the main sources of fat in the typical American diet. Unlike the healthy fats that were described in the preceding section (found primarily in vegetable sources such as raw seeds and nuts, leafy green vegetables and fish), these fats are derived from saturated fat sources. When used in excess, they contribute to such common health problems as heart disease, cancer, obesity and arthritis. Unfortunately, 40 percent (rather than the ideal 20-25 percent) of the calories in the American diet come from unhealthy, red meat-derived saturated fats.

Saturated fat tends to increase the cholesterol levels in the blood, particularly the high-risk, low-density lipoproteins that initiate the plaque formation in the blood vessels. Plaque formation can eventually lead to heart attacks and strokes. In contrast, the "good" fats derived from fish and vegetable sources can prevent heart attacks by reducing the tendency for the blood to clot. A high-saturated fat diet can also lead to obesity in women of all ages. Menopausal women are particularly at risk because their metabolism slows down with age and they burn calories less efficiently. One gram of fat contains nine calories versus the four calories contained in one gram of protein or carbohydrate. As a result, fatty foods are much higher in calories per unit weight. Although saturated fats do provide the body with a concentrated source of energy, very few of us need these extra calories. Instead of burning the fat for energy, we tend to store it in our cells as excess poundage.

As mentioned earlier, a high-fat, low-fiber diet is also associated with colon cancer, prostate cancer in men, and some breast cancer in women. In a study published in the *Journal of the National Cancer Institute*, 2,300 volunteers were examined as to their dietary habits with emphasis on their fat and oil intake. Women with breast cancer were found to have diets high in animal fats. Women who consumed olive oil on a daily basis had a significantly lower incidence of breast cancer.

One theory concerning the correlation between saturated fat and the risk of breast cancer is that a high-fat diet promotes the conversion of estrogen metabolites by anaerobic bacteria in the intestinal tract to forms of estrogen that can be easily reabsorbed back into the body. This elevates the blood estrogen level with types of estrogen that may increase the susceptibility to breast cancer in certain women. In contrast, lowering the amount of dietary fat, while increasing the amount of high fiber foods in the diet, can help reduce the risk of hormone-dependent cancers in women.

Many American women base their meals on red meat and dairy entrees like steaks, chops, oversized meat sandwiches, and cheese sandwiches. Unfortunately, large amounts of red meat-based protein can increase the risk of osteoporosis. Protein in red meat is acidic; when a woman eats red meat in excessive amounts, her body must buffer the acid load that red meat creates. One way the body accomplishes this is by dissolving the bones. The calcium and other minerals released from the bones help restore the body's acid-alkaline balance. (This process does not occur with dairy products, which already contain calcium.)

One study comparing the incidence of osteoporosis in meat-eating women (omnivores) with that in vegetarians found a dramatic difference in bone density after age 60. Between the ages of 60 and 89, vegetarian women lost 18 percent of their bone mass, but meat-eating women lost 35 percent of their bone mass—quite a striking difference. Other studies show that the amount of protein eaten will make a difference in actual calcium levels; protein intake over three ounces a day causes loss of the calcium from the urinary tract. This has been found to be true even in low-risk groups such as young, healthy males.

Finally, red meat, dairy products and saturated oils (such as palm-kernel oil) are difficult to digest. As women age, they secrete less hydrochloric acid and fewer of the digestive enzymes needed for fat and protein breakdown in the intestinal tract. In one study, 40 percent of post menopausal women lacked hydrochloric acid. Without sufficient hydrochloric acid, red meat and other sources of protein are difficult to break down and thus, cannot be utilized properly by the body. In addition, calcium and iron absorption becomes more difficult without sufficient stomach acid.

Women who are concerned about eliminating dairy products from their diet because dairy foods are great sources of calcium can choose many other good food sources of calcium. These include nondairy milk substitutes such as rice and almond milks, beans and peas, raw seeds and nuts, green leafy vegetables, and canned salmon. Using a daily calcium supplement is probably a good idea because you are assured of receiving an optimal amount of calcium.

For optimal protein intake, your diet should emphasize whole grains, beans and peas, seeds, nuts and fish high in the beneficial Omega-3 fatty acids. It is best to eliminate red meat and dairy products or use them occasionally in small portions. A truly optimal diet for the postmenopausal woman is one with high-nutrient content, low-stress foods and easy digestibility.

Summary Chart:

Foods for Menopause Relief
Beans and peas (legumes)
Whole grains
Essential fats
Raw seeds and nuts
Green leafy vegetables
Fish
Vegetables
Fruits

Foods to Limit or Avoid
Caffeine-containing foods
Coffee
Black tea
Cola drinks
Chocolate
Alcohol
Sugar
Salt
Red meat
Dairy products
Saturated oils

13

Menus, Meal Plans & Recipes

Proper meal planning is very important if your goal is to use dietary measures to relieve and prevent menopausal symptoms without the use of estrogen replacement therapy. However, even if you are currently using hormonal therapy, a good menopause-relief diet should be followed for its general health benefits. The high-nutrient content of meals designed for menopause relief, as well as their lack of high-stress ingredients such as saturated fats and sugar, helps prevent many of the diseases that become increasingly common after midlife, such as heart disease, cancer, arthritis and diabetes mellitus.

As mentioned in the previous chapter, menopausal symptoms are much less common and tend to be milder in intensity in countries outside the United States; for example, the Japanese follow dietary practices that are quite different from the American diet. Societies with a low incidence of menopausal symptoms tend to eat a diet based on vegetable protein or fish with lots of unrefined fiber. In contrast, the American diet is based on the use of milk, egg and meat protein as well as refined flour, sugar and other stressful ingredients. These foods are usually favored over whole fruits, vegetables, grains and other highly nutritious foods.

While you do not have to eat foods from other cultures (which might taste strange and unfamiliar) to be free from menopausal symptoms, some simple dietary modifications will make a major difference in your health. In this chapter I have included many helpful menopause-relieving menus and recipes you can add to your roster. Over the years, these meal planning guidelines have helped many of my patients implement their own self-help programs. Their feedback has been very positive. Many patients have noted an immediate difference in their health and well-being and found the new foods delicious and satisfying. I hope these dietary suggestions will be helpful to you, too.

General Guidelines

Before discussing the actual meal plans, consider three principles that make the transition process easier.

Make Dietary Changes Gradually

Make the transition to a healthful menopause-relief diet in an easy and non-stressful manner. Don't try to change all your dietary habits at one time by making a clean sweep of your refrigerator and pantry. Instead, substitute several healthy foods for high-stress foods you have been eating. To do this, periodically review the lists of foods to limit and those to emphasize. Each time you review this list, pick several foods you are willing to eliminate and several to try. Review these lists as often as you choose, but try to do it on a regular basis. Every small change you make in your diet will help.

Simple and Easy-to-Prepare Meals

Many women lead busy, active lives and don't have time to cook complicated meals. For that reason, my meal plans are quick and simple to prepare, with the main emphasis on foods that are delicious and high in nutrition. For those who are accustomed to eating quick meals at fast-food restaurants or commercial snack food that is high in fat, sugar and food additives, these simple meals offer a much healthier alternative.

Guidelines for Your Own Creations

Use these menus and recipes as a starting point to create your own meal plans and food combinations. Adapt your favorite dishes using the ideas contained in this chapter so that your meals are healthful rather than harmful.

Breakfast Menus

Breakfast is the most important meal of the day. Unfortunately, many women skip breakfast entirely, which can increase menopause-related fatigue, nervousness and mood swings. Other women fall into the American habit of grabbing fast foods in the morning. They eat doughnuts, pastries and coffee in hopes of getting quick energy; instead, these foods can increase menopause-related nervous tension and irritability. Others may eat hearty breakfasts full of high-stress foods—sausages, bacon, milk, toast and butter. The high fat and salt content of these foods further stress the body and impair your health.

The healthy breakfast plan includes beverages, fruits and whole-grain foods. It also contains essential fatty acids and phytoestrogens such as flaxseed and soy products.

Luckily, breakfast has been one of the easiest meals for my patients to restructure along healthier lines. You probably eat breakfast at home alone or with family members. It tends to be a smaller and simpler meal. You may want to make healthy dietary changes in your breakfast first and then move on to lunch and dinner.

The easy-to-prepare menus in this section provide a variety of healthful and delicious breakfast meals. They can also act as guidelines for you to create your own meal plans. Recipes for foods marked with an asterisk are included later in this chapter.

Breakfast Menus

Flax shake*
Rice cakes with sesame-tofu spread*

Nondairy milk breakfast shake*
Bran muffin

Instant flax cereal
Peppermint tea

Tofu cereal*
Rose hip tea

Millet cereal*
Melon
Spring water

Oatmeal banana cereal*
Roasted grain beverage (coffee substitute)

Oatmeal maple cereal*
Chamomile tea

Whole grain toast
Sesame-tofu spread*
Apple
Mint tea

Corn muffin with flax oil
Strawberries
Orange juice

Rice cakes
Raw sesame butter and fruit preserves
Sliced grapefruit
Spring water

Lunch and Dinner Menus

These lunch and dinner menus give you a variety of ways to organize your meals. A healthy menopause program combines a variety of soups, salads, sandwiches, fresh fruits, vegetables, legumes (beans and peas) and starches, as well as one-dish combination plates, and preferably fish if meat protein is to be used. If you include red meat in your meals, these items should be used in small amounts, preferably as a garnish for a vegetarian-based meal. Try the meals in this section instead of the heavy meat and cheese-centered dishes that form the nucleus of so many fast foods and deli offerings. They are high in unhealthy saturated fats, salt and excessive calories. Recipes for foods marked with an asterisk are included later in this chapter.

Soup Menus

Lentil-tofu-rice soup*
Tomato and cucumber salad
Whole grain bread

Tomato soup
Kasha*
Rye bread with flax oil
Banana

Creamy carrot soup*
Broccoli with lemon*
Baked potato and flax oil*
Banana

Split pea-tofu soup*
Cole slaw
Applesauce

Vegetable soup
Tuna sandwich
Apple slices

One-Dish Vegetarian Meals

Pasta with flax oil and garlic*
Mixed green salad

Vegetarian tacos*
Low-salt salsa

Tofu and almond stir fry*
Steamed rice

Hummus and tahini*
Rye bread
Raw carrot and celery sticks

Rice and tofu tabouli*
Black olives
Sliced tomatoes

Two-bean dish*
Romaine lettuce salad
Whole grain bread

Salad Meals

Spinach salad
Corn muffins and flax oil

Beet salad
Rye bread with flax spread

Tofu-wild rice salad*
Sliced tomatoes

Brown rice and tofu salad*
Apple and banana slices

Apple and walnut salad
Rice cakes with sesame-tofu spread*

Fish and Poultry Meals

Poached salmon*
Brown rice
Steamed carrots*

Broiled trout*
Baked potato with flax oil*
Steamed artichoke

Broiled tuna
Mixed green salad
Broccoli with lemon*

Grilled chicken
Sliced tomatoes and cucumber
Steamed red potatoes
Green beans and almonds*

Roasted turkey breast
Brown rice
Green beans and almonds*
Cole slaw

Recipes

Flax Shake   Serves 2

2-4 tablespoons raw ground flaxseeds
1 banana
1½ cups nondairy milk
1 tablespoon of vegetarian (soy- or rice-based) protein powder

Place the ground flaxseeds in a blender. Add the remaining ingredients and blend. This recipe is high in essential fatty acids, calcium, magnesium and potassium, necessary for healthy bones and heart function, as well as stabilizing one's mood.

Non-Dairy Milk Breakfast Shake   Serves 2

2 cups nondairy milk (soy or other base)
2 tablespoons vegetarian protein powder
3 tablespoons flax oil
1 large banana
¾ cup berries (strawberries, boysenberries, blueberries or raspberries)

Combine all ingredients in a blender. Blend until smooth and serve. This delicious, creamy shake is high in essential fatty acids, phytoestrogens, vitamin C and calcium, all important nutrients for menopausal women.

Instant Flax Cereal   Serves 1

4 tablespoons raw ground flaxseeds
½-1 cup nondairy vanilla milk
½ banana, sliced
sweetener (to taste)

Place ground flaxseed in a cereal bowl and slowly add the nondairy milk, stirring the mixture together. The flax mixture will thicken into a texture like cream of rice or oatmeal. Top the cereal with sliced bananas. Add sweetener if desired. Eat the mixture right away; flaxseeds are sensitive to light, air and temperature. This cereal should be eaten cold, without cooking.

Tofu Cereal   Serves 2

4 ounces soft tofu
2 ounces nondairy vanilla milk
2 tablespoons flax oil
1 banana
½ apple (optional)
12-15 raw almonds
sweetener (if desired)

Combine all ingredients in a food processor. Blend until creamy. Pour into a bowl and serve. This is a helpful cereal for menopausal women, high in essential fatty acids, calcium, magnesium and potassium.

Millet Cereal   Serves 2

1 cup millet

2 cups water

1-2 tablespoons flaxseed oil

4 ounces nondairy milk, vanilla (soy or other base)

1 tablespoon honey

1 tablespoon raw sunflower seeds

1 tablespoon raw sesame seeds

Wash millet with cold water. Bring water to a boil and add millet. Turn heat to low, cover and cook without stirring for 20 to 30 minutes, until millet is soft. Spoon into serving bowls and add the remaining ingredients. Mix and serve. Raw sunflower and sesame seeds are excellent sources of essential fatty acids, calcium, magnesium and potassium, important nutrients for menopausal women.

Oatmeal Banana Cereal   Serves 2

⅔ cup oats

1½ cups water

2 tablespoons ground, raw flaxseeds

¼–½ cup nondairy milk, vanilla flavored

½ banana

2 teaspoons honey or brown rice syrup

Boil water in a pot. Stir in oats and return to a boil. Reduce heat to medium-low. Cook uncovered for 5 minutes, stirring occasionally. Remove from heat; let stand a few minutes. Stir in ground raw flaxseeds followed by nondairy milk and honey.

Oatmeal Maple Cereal   **Serves 2**

⅔ cup oats
1½ cups water
3 tablespoons flax oil
2 teaspoons maple syrup

Boil water in a pot; stir in oats. Return mixture to a boil; reduce heat to medium-low. Cook uncovered for 5 minutes, stirring occasionally, adding more water if needed. Remove from heat and let stand for a few minutes. Stir in flax oil and maple syrup

Sesame-Tofu Spread   **Makes 1½ cups**

¼ cup soft tofu
¼ cup raw sesame butter
¼ cup honey

Combine all ingredients in a blender. Use as a spread with rice cakes or crackers.

Split Pea-Tofu Soup   **Serves 4**

1 cup split peas
½ cup diced firm tofu
½ onion, chopped
1 small carrot, sliced
5 cups water or vegetable broth
¼ to ½ teaspoons sea salt or salt substitute

Wash peas. Place peas, chopped onions and carrots in a pot. Add the water or broth. Bring to a boil, then turn heat to low and cover pot. Cook for 45 minutes. Add sea salt and tofu. Continue to cook until peas are soft. Soup may be cooled and then pureed in a blender if you prefer a creamy texture.

Lentil-Tofu-Rice Soup   Serves 4

1 cup lentils
½ cup diced firm tofu
½ cup cooked brown rice
½ onion, chopped
½ cup carrots, chopped
5-6 cups water or vegetable broth
1 teaspoon brown rice miso

Wash lentils. Place lentils, onion, carrots, water and miso in a pot. Bring to a boil, then turn heat to low, cover pot and simmer for 45 minutes or until lentils are soft. Vary the amount of water depending on the desired thickness of the soup.

Creamy Carrot Soup   Serves 4

4 cups carrots, peeled and sliced
1¼ cups onions, diced
½ cup sweet red pepper
4 cups vegetable broth
1½ tablespoons ginger root, grated
1½ cup nondairy milk, regular or vanilla flavored

Combine carrots, onions, red peppers, vegetable broth and ginger in a large pot; cook for a half hour or until carrots are tender. Strain the vegetables and puree in a food processor. Add broth and nondairy milk to blender and puree together. Return soup to cooking pot. Cook on low for five minutes.

Tofu-Wild Rice Salad   Serves 4

6 ounces tofu
2 cups cooked wild rice
3 scallions, chopped
¼ to ½ cup minced parsley
½ green pepper, minced
Herbal oil and vinegar dressing

Cut tofu into bite-size pieces. Combine with all the other ingredients in a bowl. Mix with your favorite herbal oil-and-vinegar dressing to taste.

Note: Brown rice may be substituted for wild rice.

Brown Rice and Tofu Salad   Serves 4

2 cups cooked brown rice
4 ounces diced firm tofu
1 green onion, diced
¼ cup raisins
1½ ounces chopped almonds
¼ cup peas, cooked
¼ cup green pepper
¼ cup celery

Combine all ingredients in a bowl. The salad may be dressed with a vinaigrette dressing or with a dressing made by combining 1½ tablespoons seasoned rice wine vinegar, ½ teaspoon Worcestershire sauce, and 2½ tablespoons mayonnaise.

Kasha   Serves 4

1 cup kasha (buckwheat groats)
3-3¼ cups water
pinch sea salt

Bring ingredients to a boil, lower heat and simmer for 25 minutes, or until soft. The grains should be fluffy like rice. Buckwheat is an excellent source of bioflavonoids, an important phytoestrogen for menopausal women.

Baked Sweet Potato   Serves 4

4 sweet potatoes
1 tablespoon vegetable oil
1 tablespoon flax oil for each potato

Preheat oven to 400°F. Wash the potatoes, poke a few holes in them, and rub them with vegetable oil. Bake for 45 to 60 minutes, or until soft when pierced with a fork. Garnish with flax oil. Honey, maple syrup or chopped raw pecans may also be used. Sweet potatoes are an excellent source of beta-carotene. A diet high in beta-carotene containing foods helps reduce the incidence of breast cancer.

Baked Potato   Serves 4

4 russet or Idaho potatoes
1 tablespoon vegetable oil
1 tablespoon flax oil for each potato

Preheat oven to 400°F. Wash the potatoes, poke a few holes in them, and rub them with vegetable oil, and bake for 45 to 60 minutes, or until soft when pierced with a fork. Garnish with flax oil. Other garnishes can include chopped green onions or soy cheese. Potatoes are delicious to use with essential fatty acids like flax oil. They are also easy to digest and good sources of nutrients like vitamin C.

Steamed Kale   **Serves 4**

1 bunch kale (stems removed), chopped
Juice of 1 lemon
1-2 tablespoons olive oil
pinch of sea salt

Steam the kale until tender. Dress with lemon juice, olive oil and sea salt. Kale is a very good source of calcium for menopausal women, since the calcium contained in kale absorbs and assimilates well.

Broccoli with Lemon   **Serves 4**

1 pound broccoli
½ lemon, juiced
4 tablespoons flax oil

Cut the broccoli into small flowerets; steam for 6 minutes, or until tender. Squeeze lemon juice over the broccoli and add the flax oil. Mix and serve. For an exciting taste treat try substituting Bragg's Liquid Amino Acids for the juiced lemon. Broccoli is a good source of calcium and magnesium, important nutrients for healthy bones. It is also high in vitamin A and other nutrients thought to confer protection against cancer.

Steamed Carrots   **Serves 4**

8 medium carrots, sliced
1 tablespoon maple syrup

Steam carrots until soft. Top with maple syrup and serve. Carrots are an excellent source of beta-carotene, an important nutrient for cancer protection.

Green Beans and Almonds   Serves 4

1 pound green beans
2 ounces raw almonds, chopped
2 tablespoons flax oil
¼ teaspoon sea salt

Steam green beans until tender. Toss with the chopped almond, flax oil and sea salt for a buttery flavor. If you don't care for the taste of flax oil, a vinaigrette may be substituted. Flax oil may also be used to dress a variety of other vegetables.

Rice and Tofu Tabouli   Serves 6

2 cups cooked brown rice
¼-½ cup parsley, chopped
½ cup fresh mint, chopped
¼ medium red onion, diced
1 medium tomato, diced
2 ounces firm tofu, diced
1 lemon, juiced
2 tablespoons olive oil
¼ teaspoon sea salt
1 teaspoon cumin
1 teaspoon oregano

Place rice in a bowl. Mix in parsley, mint, red onion, tomato, and diced tofu. Combine these ingredients thoroughly. Add lemon juice and olive oil and mix. Add cumin, oregano and salt to the salad and mix well. This is the ultimate delicious and healthy tabouli recipe. It is great served with the hummus and tahini recipe described below.

Hummus and Tahini   Makes 2 cups

3 tablespoons raw, sesame tahini
1¾-2 cups garbanzo beans, cooked
1 clove of raw garlic
3 tablespoons lemon juice
¼ teaspoon salt
water as needed

Combine water, garbanzo beans, sesame tahini, lemon juice, olive oil, garlic and salt in a food processor. Blend to the consistency of a smooth dip. Serve as a dip with gluten free bread, rye bread and fresh vegetables. This dip is an excellent source of essential fatty acids, calcium and easy to digest vegetable protein.

Two-Bean Dish   Serves 2

¾ cup black beans, cooked
¾ cup lentils or great northern beans, cooked
¼ red pepper, diced
¼ small red onion, diced
2 ounces celery, diced
1 cup brown rice
6 leaves romaine lettuce
2 tablespoons chopped green onions
oil and vinegar

In two separate bowls, combine each bean portion with half the red pepper, red onion and celery. Mix well. On a serving dish arrange leaves of romaine lettuce. Place the cup of brown rice in the center and arrange beans on either side. Sprinkle with chopped green onions and dress with oil and vinegar or your favorite vinaigrette dressing. Beans are an excellent source of calcium as well as easy-to-digest vegetable protein.

Pasta with Flax Oil and Garlic   Serves 4

1 pound pasta
2-3 garlic cloves, minced
4 tablespoons flax oil
1 tablespoon soy Parmesan cheese (available at health food stores)
1 teaspoon basil
½ teaspoon sea salt

Cook pasta until tender. Top with garlic, flax oil, basil, salt and soy parmesan. Mix until well blended and serve.

Tofu and Almond Stir Fry   Serves 4

¾ cups firm tofu, cubed
¼-½ cup raw almonds, chopped
½ red pepper, chopped
¼ yellow onion, chopped
¼ cup water
1 teaspoon sesame or safflower oil
3 cups brown rice, cooked
1 teaspoon wheat-free soy sauce

Combine tofu, almonds, onions and red peppers in a large frying pan with oil, add a small amount of water if necessary. Cook over low flame for 5 minutes. Add rice to pan and mix. Cook for 5 minutes or until warm. Transfer to serving dish and toss with wheat-free soy sauce.

Vegetarian Tacos   **Serves 4**

4-8 corn tortillas
1 can pinto beans
1 cup brown rice
1 avocado, thinly sliced
¼ red onion, finely chopped
¼ sweet red pepper, diced
1 tomato, diced
½ cup salsa, or to taste
1-2 cups red or romaine lettuce, chopped

Warm tortillas and beans in separate pans. Place tortillas on individual serving dishes and spread with beans and rice. Garnish with avocado, pepper, tomato, lettuce and onion. Serve with salsa.

Poached Salmon   **Serves 4**

4 fillets of salmon, 3 ounces each
1 cup water
1 lemon

Combine water and juice of one lemon in skillet and heat. Place the salmon in the hot liquid and cook on medium or medium-low heat. Cover and poach for 6 to 8 minutes, or until the salmon flakes easily with a fork. Remove the fish and keep it warm until ready to serve.

Broiled Trout   **Serves 4**

2 fresh trout fillets, 6-8 ounces each
2 tablespoons lemon juice
chopped fresh dill (dried if fresh is unavailable)

Slice each fillet in half. This will make four servings of trout. Sprinkle the fillets with lemon juice and dill. Place the trout in a broiler pan. Broil for 5 to 6 minutes, or until done.

Substitute Healthy Ingredients in Recipes

Many of the recipes you have now probably contain ingredients that women with menopausal symptoms should avoid, such as caffeine, alcohol, sugar, chocolate, and dairy products. Learning how to make substitutions for high-stress ingredients in familiar recipes allows you to make your favorite foods without compromising your emotional or physical health.

Some women choose to totally eliminate high-stress ingredients from a recipe. For example, you can make a pasta dish with tomato sauce but eliminate the Parmesan cheese topping and use non-wheat pasta. Greek salad can be made without the feta cheese. You may even make pizza substituting soy cheese, layering tomato sauce and lots of vegetables on the crust. In many cases, the high-stress ingredients are not necessary to make foods taste good; always remember, they can make your anxiety symptoms worse and impair your health.

If you want to use a particular high-stress ingredient, you can usually substantially reduce the amount of that ingredient you use, while still retaining the flavor and taste. Most of us have palates jaded by too much fat, salt, sugar and other flavorings. In many dishes, we taste only the additives; we never really enjoy the delicious flavors of the foods themselves. Now that I regularly substitute low-stress ingredients in my cooking, I enjoy the subtle taste of the dishes much more, and my health and vitality continue to improve. The following information tells you how to easily substitute healthy ingredients in your own recipes.

Caffeinated Foods and Beverages

Drink substitutes for coffee and black tea. The best substitutes are the grain-based coffee beverages, such as Postum and Cafix. Some women may find the abrupt discontinuance of coffee difficult because of withdrawal symptoms, such as headaches. If this concerns you, decrease your total coffee intake gradually to one or one-half cup per day. Use coffee substitutes for your other cups. This will help prevent withdrawal symptoms.

Use decaffeinated coffee or tea as a transition beverage. If you cannot give up coffee, start by substituting water-processed decaffeinated coffee for the real thing. Then try to wean yourself from coffee altogether or go to a coffee substitute. You can also get ginger tea bags at most health food stores.

Use herbal teas for energy and vitality. Many women with anxiety and the excessive stress that may accompany menopause mistakenly drink coffee as a pick me up to be able to function during the day. Use ginger tea instead. It is a great herbal stimulant that won't damage your health. To make ginger tea, grate a few teaspoons of fresh ginger root into a pot of hot water; boil and steep. Serve with honey.

Substitute carob for chocolate. Unsweetened carob tastes like chocolate but doesn't contain the anxiety-causing caffeine found in chocolate. A member of the legume family, carob is high in calcium. You can purchase it in chunk form as a substitute for chocolate candy or as a powder for use in baking or drinks. Be careful, however, not to overindulge; carob, like chocolate, is high in calories and fat. Consider it a treat and an excellent cooking aid for use in small amounts only.

Sugar

Substitute concentrated sweeteners. Americans use too much sugar, which only increases symptoms of nervous tension, a problem during early menopause. I have found that as women decrease their sugar intake, most begin to enjoy the subtle flavors of the foods they eat. Concentrated sweeteners such as honey and maple syrup have a sweeter taste per quantity used than table sugar. Using these substitutes will allow you to decrease the amount of table sugar you use in a recipe. If you use a concentrated sweetener in place of sugar in the average recipe, reduce the liquid content in the recipe by one-fourth cup. If no liquid is used in the recipe, add three to five tablespoons of flour for each three-fourths cup of concentrated sweetener.

Substitute fruit for sugar in baked goods. When making muffins and cookies, you may want to try substituting sugar with extra fruits, nuts, applesauce and brown rice syrup.

Alcohol

Use low alcohol or nonalcoholic products for drinking or cooking. There are many low and nonalcoholic wines and beers available in supermarkets and liquor stores. Many of these taste quite good and can be used for meals or other social occasions. In addition, you can substitute low-alcohol or nonalcoholic wine or beer when cooking or preparing sauces and marinades. You will retain much of the flavor that alcohol imparts, and you'll decrease the stress factor substantially.

Dairy Products

Eliminate or decrease the amount of cow's milk cheese you use in food preparation and cooking. If you prefer to use cow's milk cheese in cooking, decrease the amount in the recipe by three-fourths so that it becomes a flavoring or garnish rather than a major source of fat and protein. For example, use one teaspoon of Parmesan cheese on top of a casserole instead of one-half cup.

Use soy cheese in food preparation and cooking. Soy cheese is an excellent substitute for cow's milk cheese. It is often lower in fat and salt, and the fat it does contain isn't saturated. Women with severe fatigue may have difficulty digesting it, so I recommend its use only to women who do not suffer from severe fatigue. Health food stores offer many brands and flavors, such as mozzarella, cheddar, American and jack. The quality of these products keeps improving all the time. You can use soy cheese as a perfect cheese substitute in sandwiches, salads, pizzas, lasagnas and casseroles. In some recipes you can replace cheese with soft tofu. I have done this often with lasagna, layering the lasagna noodles with tofu and topping with melted soy cheese for a delicious dish.

Replace milk and yogurt in recipes. For dairy milk, substitute soy milk, nut milk or grain milk. Soy milk and nut milk are available at most health food stores. Soy milk is particularly good and comes in many flavors. Many nondairy types of milk are good sources of calcium and can be used for drinking, eating or baking. Three to four glasses of soymilk each day provides a significant amount of the phytoestrogen soy isoflavones. The higher the protein content of the milk, the more soy isoflavones it contains. Soy milk though can be difficult for some women to digest.

For dairy-based yogurt, substitute soy yogurt. Several excellent brands of soy yogurt are available in health food stores in plain, vanilla and various fruit flavors. Its great taste approximates dairy milk yogurt. Soy yogurt works well for both cooking and baking.

Substitute flax oil for butter. Flax oil is the best substitute for butter I've found: a rich, golden oil that looks and tastes like butter. It is delicious on anything you'd normally top with butter—toast, rice, popcorn, steamed vegetables or potatoes. Flax oil is extremely high in essential fatty acids— the type of fat that is very healthy for a woman's body. Essential fatty acids improve vitality, enhance circulation, and help promote normal hormonal function. Flax oil is very perishable, however, because it is sensitive to heat and light. You can't cook with it—cook the food first and add the flax oil before serving. Also, keep it refrigerated. Flax oil has so many health benefits that I highly recommend its use; it can be found in health food stores.

Red Meat

Substitute turkey, chicken, eggs, beans, tofu, or seeds in recipes. You can often modify recipes calling for red meat by substituting ground turkey, ground chicken, or tofu. For example, use ground turkey or crumble up tofu to simulate the texture of hamburger and add to recipes like enchiladas, tacos, chili, meatloaf, and ground beef casseroles. Ground turkey and ground chicken are very flavorful. The tofu takes on the flavor of the sauce used in the dish and is indistinguishable from red meat. I often do this when cooking at home.

When making salads that call for ham or bacon, such as chef's salad or Cobb salad, substitute turkey bacon and add kidney beans, garbanzo beans, hard boiled eggs, or sunflower seeds. These will provide the needed protein, yet be more healthful and, often, more easily digestible. You can also sprinkle sunflower seeds on top of casseroles for extra protein and essential fatty acids. When making stir-fries substitute turkey, chicken, tofu, almonds, or sprouts for red meat.

Use soy and wheat-based meat substitutes. For those women who want to prepare vegetarian food, yet still miss the taste and texture of meat, these products may provide the solution. Companies that produce these substitutes manufacture products that now taste astonishingly like sausage, hot dogs, ham-burger, chicken, bologna, pepperoni, and other forms of meat.

However, women who have soy and wheat allergies should avoid these substitutes and use organic, free range chicken and turkey sausages and hot dogs, free range organic beef or bison hamburgers and other healthier types of meat, instead.

Wheat Flour

Use whole grain, non-wheat flour. Wheat flour is a source of gluten, an allergenic and difficult to digest protein. Substitute whole grain, non-wheat flours, such as rice flour. Whole grain flours are much higher in essential nutrients, such as vitamin B complex and many minerals. They are also higher in fiber content. Rice flour makes excellent cookies, cakes and other pastries. Rice flour is also excellent for pie crusts.

Salt

Substitute potassium-based products for table salt (sodium chloride). Potassium-based products, such as Morton's Salt Substitute, are much healthier and will not aggravate heart disease or hypertension.

Use powdered seaweed such as kelp or non to season vegetables, grains and salads. They are high in essential iodine and trace elements.

Use herbs instead of salt for flavoring. Herbs have subtle flavors that will help even the most jaded palate appreciate the taste of fresh fruits, vegetables and meats.

Use liquid flavoring agents with advertised low-sodium content. Low-salt soy sauce and Bragg's Amino Acids, a liquid soybean-based flavoring agent, are delicious when used as salt substitutes in cooking. Add them to soups, casseroles, stir-fries and other dishes at the end of the cooking process. You need only a small amount for intense flavoring.

Substitutes for Common High-Stress Ingredients

High-Stress Ingredient	Low-Stress Substitute
¾ cup sugar	¾ cup xylitol
	½ cup honey
	¼ cup molasses
	½ cup maple syrup
	¾ cup brown rice syrup
	1 cup apple butter
	2 cups apple juice
1 cup milk	1 cup soy, rice, nut, or grain milk
1 cup yogurt	1 cup soy, rice, or other nondairy yogurt
1 tablespoon butter	1 tablespoon flax oil (must be used raw and unheated)
½ teaspoon salt	1 teaspoon miso
	½ teaspoon potassium chloride salt substitute
	½ teaspoon Mrs. Dash, Spike
	½ teaspoon herbs (basil, tarragon, oregano, etc.)
1½ cups cocoa	1 cup powdered carob
1 square chocolate	¾ tablespoon powdered carob
1 tablespoon coffee	1 tablespoon decaffeinated coffee
	1 tablespoon Postum, Cafix, or other grain-based coffee substitute
4 ounces wine	4 ounces non-alcoholic wine
8 ounces beer	8 ounces non-alcoholic beer
1 cup white flour	1 cup barley flour (pie crust)
	1 cup rice flour (cookies, cakes, breads)
1 cup meat	1 cup beans or tofu
	¼ cup seeds

14

Healthy Plant Based Sources of Estrogen

There are many foods, herbs and nutrients that replicate estrogen's role in your body. I have found that a combination of plant-based foods and nutrients, yin herbs, and key vitamins are very helpful in combating menopause symptoms in women who are estrogen deficient. These hormone substitutes provide a safe, estrogen-like effect. Using them in a combination that works best for you on a regular basis, in sufficient amounts, can improve your hormone status and greatly reduce menopause symptoms.

Estrogen Support with Phyto Foods

Flaxseeds

Essential fatty acids are critical for health and must be supplied daily by the diet, as the body cannot make them. The skin is full of fatty acids that, along with estrogen, provide moisture, softness, and smooth texture. When estrogen levels decline with menopause, moisture can continue to be provided to tissues of the skin, vagina, and bladder, as well as the hair, by increasing the intake of fatty acid containing foods. Excellent sources of essential fatty acids are fish, nuts, and seeds, especially **flaxseeds.** Flaxseeds are particularly good for skin and hair dryness that many women experience once they enter menopause.

Both ground whole flaxseeds, which are 30 percent oil by content, and cold-pressed organic flaxseed oil used as a food supplement, are excellent sources of the two essential oils, alpha-linolenic acid and linoleic acid. Flaxseed is unusual since it also contains a double source of plant-based estrogen. Both the oil and the flax lignan (a substance contained within the cellulose like material that provides structure to plants) contained within the seed have been researched for their weakly estrogenic effect.

A study published in the *British Medical Journal* described how shifting the diet toward phytoestrogen-containing foods can change certain menopause indicators. In this study, twenty-five menopausal women (average age: fifty-nine) were asked to supplement their normal diet with phytoestrogen-containing foods such as flaxseed oil. The women consumed these foods over a six-week period. Smears from the vaginal wall were taken every two weeks to see if the addition of estrogen-containing plant foods would cause a beneficial hormonal effect on the vagina. Typically, the vaginal mucosa thins out and becomes more prone to trauma and infections as the estrogen level drops with menopause. Interestingly, the vaginal mucosa responded significantly to the additional ingestion of flaxseed oil and soy flour but returned to previous levels eight weeks after these foods were discontinued and the women went back to their usual diet.

Seeds and whole grains also contain lignans, which make up part of the structure of plants. Once plant lignans are eaten, intestinal bacteria convert them to substances that are weakly estrogenic and can provide additional nutritional support to menopausal women deficient in this hormone. This was confirmed in a study appearing in *Proceedings of the Society for Experimental Biology and Medicine*. Flaxseeds are 100 times richer in lignans than any other plant. Other sources of essential fatty acids include evening primrose oil, borage oil, and black currant oil. Unlike flaxseed oil, these other oils are not used as foods, but as nutritional supplements.

For women who are still having periods, flaxseed can act as a menstrual regulator. In a study conducted at the University of Minnesota, published in the *Journal of Clinical Endocrinology and Metabolism*, eighteen women with normal menstrual cycles ate normally for three cycles and then added 10 g of flaxseed powder per day to their diet for an additional three cycles. During the time that the women did not eat flaxseed, there were three cycles when no ovulation occurred. But when flaxseed was included, all of the women in the study ovulated every menstrual cycle. Thus, ground flaxseed was found to improve the estrogen-to-progesterone ratio favoring the levels of progesterone within the body. Progesterone production occurs only in ovulatory menstrual cycles.

Another very important benefit of ground flaxseed is that research studies have shown that it provides protection against breast cancer in women and, even, prostate cancer in men. Research studies in postmenopausal women with breast cancer found that flaxseed lignans reduce the growth and aggressiveness of the tumors and even enhance tumor death and destruction when fed muffins containing flaxseed. Women who were fed placebos- muffins without the flaxseed- did not show any of these benefits against breast. Research studies have shown similar benefits on prostate cancer in men who have been diagnosed with this disease.

Our skin is filled with fatty acids that, along with estrogen, provide the moisture, softness, and smooth texture that we prize in beautiful and healthy looking skin. When our estrogen levels decline with menopause, we can continue to provide moisture to the skin, vagina, and bladder mucosa by increasing levels of essential fatty acid-containing foods. Flaxseed oil is particularly good for dry skin since it contains high levels of both of the major essential fatty acids. In addition, fatty acids are a main structural component of all cell membranes and are found in high levels in such important tissues as the brain and nerve cells, adrenal gland, retina, and inner ear.

Besides relieving tissue dryness, the essential fatty acids found in flaxseed are needed by the body as precursors for the production of important hormone-like chemicals called prostaglandins. Body tissues manufacture over thirty types of prostaglandins. The proper balance of prostaglandins can play a major role in relieving and preventing many diseases that occur predominantly in the postmenopausal period.

For example, beneficial prostaglandins keep the platelets, a component of blood, from sticking or clumping together. This reduces the likelihood of heart attacks and strokes by preventing clotting of the blood and obstruction of the blood vessels. Since the incidence of heart attacks increases tenfold between the ages of fifty-five and sixty-five, this can benefit women who are in the postmenopausal period. In addition, they reduce inflammation, and thus the symptoms of arthritis. Many women date the onset of arthritis symptoms after menopause. Beneficial prostaglandins also stimulate immune function and helps insulin to function effectively.

Flaxseed oil is sold in opaque containers in the refrigerator section of most health food stores, as it is very sensitive to heat, light, and oxygen. Flaxseed oil bottles are dated to ensure that they are used quickly to preserve their freshness. Flaxseed oil can even be stored in the freezer, as can seeds and nuts, until you are ready to use them. It is also marketed as a ground meal and in capsule form.

I recommend substituting flaxseed oil for butter. Flaxseed oil is the best substitute for butter that I've found. It is a rich, golden oil that looks and tastes quite a bit like butter. It is delicious on anything you'd normally top with butter—toast, rice, popcorn, steamed vegetables, or potatoes. Flaxseed oil is extremely high in essential fatty acids—the type of fat that is very healthy for a woman's body. Essential fatty acids improve vitality, enhance circulation, and help promote healthy hormonal function. Flaxseed oil is quite perishable, however, because it is sensitive to heat and light. For that reason, don't cook with it—cook the food first and add the flaxseed oil before serving. Also, keep it refrigerated even before opening it. Because flaxseed oil has so many health benefits, I highly recommend its use. You can find it in most health food stores.

Ground flax meal, which contains the whole seed, is also available in health food stores. It can be stirred into hot cereal like oatmeal or used in shakes and smoothies. It is an excellent source of fiber as well as phytoestrogens. Like flaxseed oil, it needs to be refrigerated to maintain its freshness. **I recommend taking 1 to 2 tablespoons of flaxseed oil each day or 2 to 4 tablespoons of ground flax meal.**

Laura's Story

When Laura came to see me, she was in her mid-50's. She had been struggling with menopause-related symptoms for nearly two years, and every attempt at hormone replacement therapy had ended in frustration. Her doctor had put her on two different types of conventional hormone replacement therapy (HRT)—Premarin (an estrogen combination) and Provera (a progestin). However, both gave her very unpleasant side effects.

She eventually quit taking conventional HRT altogether and started using black cohosh and vitamin E. While these natural remedies didn't cause any of the negative side effects she had experienced with HRT, they weren't very effective in relieving her symptoms.

I quickly realized she was taking the wrong dosages. I got her on the proper doses of these supplements so that they would be more effective in controlling here symptoms. I also realized that her diet needed attention. She had a very low quality diet, full of refined foods, sugar and fat. Too many cups of coffee each day and several glasses of wine each night were contributing to her hot flashes and insomnia.

I recommended that she eliminate these high stress foods and also that she begin eating a high phytoestrogen diet including ground flax meal in her cereal each day and cultured soy yogurt, which she really liked. She was very pleased to notice that her symptoms began to diminish significantly.

Pomegranate

Super fruits like pomegranate are a rich source of antioxidants like polyphenols, some of which have anti-inflammatory benefits. Pomegranates also contain a high content of anthocyanins which are a subcategory of plant bioflavonoids. These are the pigments that give these fruits their strong, beautiful colors like reds and purples and are also protective antioxidants.

In case you don't know what an antioxidant is, let me explain. An antioxidant is a substance that protects our bodies from free radical damage. A free radical is a type of oxygen molecule that freely moves inside cells, reacting with proteins, fats, and DNA, changing and damaging their structure and disrupting their functions. Free radicals are generated by the metabolism of oxygen and other chemicals, including cigarette smoke, unsaturated fats, food additives, and environmental chemicals—and even by aerobic exercise. Free radicals can cause an extreme amount of damage within our bodies.

Antioxidants help to protect us from free radical damage. Antioxidants unite with free radicals and deactivate them, preventing them from doing damage. A variety of substances have an antioxidant function, including vitamin C, vitamin A, beta-carotene, vitamin E, selenium, and glutathione. It is important to either include all of the antioxidants in the diet or take them as supplements.

There are also specific benefits for women in eating pomegranates. They contain natural plant estrogens which may be useful in relieving vaginal dryness, supporting bone health and balancing mood in menopausal women. According to a study published in *Cancer Prevention Research* and reported by the Cleveland Clinic, substances found in pomegranate may help prevent estrogen dependent breast cancers. Pomegranates contain polyphenols called ellagitannins that are converted to urolithin A and B in the intestines. These substances block an enzyme called aromatase that converts androgen (male hormones) to estrogen, which stimulates certain breast cancers.

Pomegranate has other health benefits. Early research on pomegranate juice suggests that it may improve blood flow to the heart is people with coronary heart disease as well as improve the lipid profile in diabetic patients. Research on kidney dialysis patients found that pomegranate juice reduced inflammation and kidney damage. According to research done at UCLA, It may also be beneficial in slowing the growth of prostate cancer. **I recommend taking 500 mg capsules of pomegranate extract, once or twice a day. You can also drink pomegranate juice which is less desirable because of its fruit sugar content.**

Soybean Isoflavones

Many research studies have confirmed that soybean-based products can actually help reduce and prevent menopause symptoms. Soybeans are filled with natural plant estrogens (or phytoestrogens) called isoflavones. Weak estrogenic activity is found in a variety of plant foods and herbs. However, for therapeutic purposes, only soybeans contain sufficient active compounds to approximate the effects of estrogen produced by the body. Soy contains two main phytoestrogens—genistein and daidzein, which belong to the class of chemicals called isoflavones.

Soy isoflavones were first discovered during the 1930s, but their potency was not assayed until the 1950s. At that time, genistein was found to be 50,000 times weaker than a powerful synthetic estrogen. Asian women eat much more soy products in their traditional diet than American women, whose isoflavone intake is virtually zero. This was confirmed in a study published in *The Lancet*, which found that Japanese women who regularly eat a range of soy products had 100 to 1,000 times more isoflavone breakdown products in their urine than Western women. Additionally, menopausal women in Japan are rarely troubled by symptoms such as hot flashes.

As weak estrogens, these compounds bind to estrogen receptors and act as a substitute form of estrogen in the body. They compete with the more potent estrogens made by a woman's body for these cell receptor sites. As a result, isoflavones can help to regulate estrogen levels.

High estrogen levels can worsen female problems like heavy menstrual flow, PMS, fibroid tumors of the uterus, endometriosis, and fibrocystic breast lumps. A soy-based diet can decrease the severity of these problems by reducing the toxic effects of the more potent estrogens made within our bodies on estrogen-sensitive tissues like the breast and uterus.

After menopause, when estrogen levels can become deficient, dietary sources of estrogen such as soy can provide much-needed hormonal support for the body. In fact, a diet high in isoflavone-rich soybeans can actually reduce the incidence of menopause symptoms. Asian women eat much more soy products in their traditional diet than American women, whose isoflavone intake is virtually zero. This was confirmed in a study published in *The Lancet*, which found that Japanese women who regularly eat a range of soy products had 100 to 1,000 times more isoflavone breakdown products in their urine than Western women.

In Japan only 10 to 15 percent of the women experience menopause symptoms. By contrast, 80 to 85 percent of women in the United States, Canada, and Europe who eat a traditional Western diet experience menopausal symptoms.

One study reported in the *British Medical Journal* examined how shifting the diet towards phytoestrogen-containing foods can change certain menopause indicators. In this study, 25 menopausal women (average age fifty-nine) were asked to supplement their normal diet with phytoestrogen containing foods like soy flour, flaxseed oil, and red clover sprouts. The women consumed these foods over a six-week period, each food for two weeks at a time.

Smears of the vaginal wall were taken every week to see if the addition of estrogen-containing plant foods would cause a beneficial hormonal effect on the vagina. (Typically, the vaginal mucosa thins out and becomes more prone to trauma and infections as the estrogen level drops with menopause.) Interestingly, the vaginal mucosa did respond significantly to the intake of soy flour and flaxseed oil (not to the red clover sprouts) but returned to its previous state eight weeks after these foods were discontinued and the women went back to their normal diets. Studies have also shown the benefit of soybeans in reducing hot flashes.

Other research studies have measured phytoestrogen excretion, comparing groups with a diet rich in soy and other phytoestrogens to groups eating the typical Western omnivorous diet. One study showed that men, women, and children in Japan and America who ate a diet high in soy foods like tofu, boiled soybeans, and miso excreted 100 to 1000 times more beneficial isoflavones in their urine than women in Finland and the United States who ate a meat and dairy-based diet. In fact, isoflavone content tends to be eighty percent lower in the typical American or European meat and dairy-based diet, than it is in a plant-based diet.

Although this has been the subject of controversy, research studies are more aligned with the findings that isoflavones found in soybeans have the added benefit of being anti-carcinogenic. Research has linked a high intake of soybean-based foods to the lower incidence of breast cancer and lower mortality from prostate cancer among Japanese women and men, respectively. Research studies done in the U.S. have confirmed the benefits of soy foods for prostate cancer. Other clinical studies have found that soy helps to lower cholesterol levels, thereby helping to reduce the incidence of heart attacks.

Soy is available in many forms in the United States. Tofu, an inexpensive, bland, curd-like soy product, can be found in most supermarkets and health food stores. Tofu will take on the flavor of any food that you cook it with, which makes it an ideal source of protein and essential fatty acids that you can add to soups, stir-fries, casseroles, and other dishes. Tempeh is a cultured soy product made of the whole soybean. Besides being a good source of protein, it contains vitamin B12, a nutrient needed for the production of healthy blood cells and nerve function. Purely vegetarian diets are often deficient in vitamin B12. Thus, adding tempeh can be helpful. Miso is often used to make soup.

One of the most interesting uses of soy is as a dairy substitute. Any dairy is now available in a soy-based version. This includes soy milk cheese, sour cream, yogurt, cream cheese, and ice cream-like desserts. Although the soy cheeses generally tend not to be as tasty or textured as cow's milk based cheeses, they can still be used as good substitutes in recipes. Soy-based meat such as hot dogs, burgers, and other substitute meat products can be very tasty too. Be sure to look at the label of each product to make sure that it is not too high in either salt or fat.

Concerns about Soy's Side-Effects

It seems that we are bombarded on a daily basis with new information about soy—in some cases praising its benefits, and in other cases making it the scapegoat for everything from Alzheimer's to early maturation of teenage girls. While a handful of the critical studies have some merit, many are based on questionable research or test tube science. These studies really lose their impact when compared to the hundreds of clinical, animal, and epidemiological studies that attest to soy's health-protective benefits.

Still, I receive questions almost weekly about the dangers of soy and breast cancer and/or thyroid function. In my experience, I believe that it is probably safe for women with breast cancer to eat soy foods in moderation, with one caveat. In a study published in *Cancer Research,* researchers investigated the interactions between dietary genistein and tamoxifen and breast cancer by implanting estrogen-dependent breast cancer cells in mice who had had their ovaries and thymus removed. They found that genistein negated or overwhelmed the inhibitory effect of tamoxifen. Based on these findings, they urged postmenopausal women to exercise caution when consuming soy based genistein while taking tamoxifen.

To date, I have not seen anything in the literature to negate this conclusion. Therefore, if you have breast cancer and are taking tamoxifen, I suggest that you use caution and avoid using pure soy isoflavones unless further, more conclusive studies contradict these findings. However, if you have questions about the advisability of using soy foods for your particular case, I recommend that you check with your doctor.

In the case of hypothyroidism, I believe that the concern over soy's impact on thyroid function is unwarranted. First, no well-controlled, statistically significant human studies have shown that soy interferes with thyroid function. In fact, several studies conducted on humans have found no difference in thyroid function between those women who ate soy and those who did not. Second, the lack of evidence surrounding this topic has led the FDA to reverse its earlier position that soy adversely affected the thyroid. Even more compelling is the fact that the American Foundation of Thyroid Patients has reviewed the current medical literature on soy and thyroid health and now recommends soy for all its members.

Based on the research as well as my experience, I see no reason for most women with a thyroid condition to avoid soy or soy products. The only exception I have made is for women who have inflammatory bowel disease and autoimmune thyroiditis, combined with a known allergy or sensitivity to soy. For this very small group of women, I recommend avoiding soy, as it may aggravate their condition.

Eating soy-based foods also has several other long-term health benefits. Unlike prescription estrogen, soy does not appear to have a carcinogenic effect on uterine cells or breast tissue. In fact, it appears to be cancer-protective for several reasons. Not only does soy reduce the production of estrogen within the body, but it also directly inhibits the growth of breast cancer cells. A review article appearing in the *Journal of the American Dietetics Association* noted that soybean intake is associated with reduced rates of prostate, colon, and breast cancer. Once again, we see this benefit in Japanese women, who have an incidence of breast cancer four to six times lower than that of women who do not include soy in their diet.

Other studies currently in progress suggest that soy can have a beneficial effect on both blood fats and bone metabolism. While estrogen is often prescribed to prevent heart disease and osteoporosis, soy offers a food-based approach to the same health issues.

Still, soy is not for everyone. Some women don't like the taste of soy foods and other women have difficulty digesting it. It is one option among many that you can choose from to help relieve menopause symptoms.

If you are allergic to soy, then obviously you need to avoid consuming it entirely. If you find that soy foods cause digestive upset such as gas, bloating, or intestinal discomfort, I suggest taking a high-potency digestive enzyme such as bromelain or papain whenever you consume soy foods, or simply opt for supplemental soy isoflavones capsules.

I recommend that you take in 50–100 mg of soy isoflavones each day, either through soy foods or isoflavone capsules, or a combination of both.

Isoflavones in Soy Foods

Whole soybeans (edamame) — 150 mg
Soy milk — 35–40 mg
Tempeh — 35 mg
Tofu — 35 mg

Kathleen's Story

When Kathleen first consulted with me, she had a busy career, lived on unhealthy but convenient fast food meals, and was 25 pounds overweight. She was postmenopausal, with high blood pressure and cholesterol. Moreover, she had lost considerable bone mass—even though she was only in her early 50s. She was very concerned about the negative direction that her health was going in and wanted to reverse this pattern.

Kathleen was a perfect candidate for soy foods. She was thrilled that she could substitute soy burgers for the high-fat, high-sodium cheeseburgers she had been eating, and started to explore other soy foods such as tofu, tempeh, soy milk, soy yogurt, and soy cheese. She also began adding healthy salads, soups, steamed vegetables, nuts, and other legumes to her diet. In addition to soy foods, I put Kathleen on a powerful program of nutritional supplements and bioidentical hormones.

She was absolutely thrilled with the results—her excess weight fell off rapidly, her blood pressure and cholesterol dropped, and her bone mineral density improved. She enjoyed her new diet so much that she became increasingly interested in cooking and experimenting with healthy recipes—something she had never done before in her life!

The Healing Power of Plants

Many herbs are estrogen like in their activity, including common culinary herbs such as fennel and anise, as well as licorice. Other herbs, such as black cohosh and red clover, have been used medicinally as part of healing traditions for thousands of years. While their estrogenic activity is a small fraction of the activity of the estrogen a woman produces (at least 400 times less active), their benefit is that these herbs usually do not cause unwanted side effects for most women.

Black Cohosh

One of the most effective estrogen supportive herbs is black cohosh. Native to America, black cohosh was well known and accepted in Native American herbal medicine and was widely prescribed in colonial times as a treatment for menstrual cramps and menopausal symptoms.

The effectiveness and safety of black cohosh are well documented. Clinical studies have shown that black cohosh relieves hot flashes, night sweats, heart palpitations, headaches, and vaginal dryness and atrophy. It is also effective in relieving other symptoms such as depression, anxiety, sleep disturbances, and a decline in libido.

Currently, in Germany, a special extract of black cohosh is the most thoroughly studied and widely used natural alternative to hormone replacement therapy. This research has prompted at least six well-publicized studies on the standardized extract of black cohosh and its ability to treat menopausal symptoms. According to a review of five key studies on black cohosh from the *American Journal of Medicine*, black cohosh is most effective at easing hot flashes.

In one of the largest studies on black cohosh, women with menopausal complaints received 40 drops of liquid black cohosh extract twice a day for six to eight weeks. Within four weeks of treatment, a distinct improvement was seen in nearly 80 percent of the women. After six to eight weeks, all symptoms had completely disappeared in half of the women.

Another study found similar results. Scientists gave women with menopausal symptoms either high or low-dose black cohosh for a 12-week period. At the conclusion of the study, approximately 80 percent of both patients and physicians rated the treatment as "good to very good." The investigators reported no differences in either effectiveness or adverse reactions between the two groups.

Other studies have focused on black cohosh and its relationship to breast cancer. One in particular concluded that black cohosh actually inhibits the growth rate of breast cancer cells due to the herb's lack of estrogen-like effects in certain breast cancer cell lines whose growth is dependent upon estrogen. Laboratory experiments have shown that black cohosh inhibits the effects of estrogen-induced stimulation and actually binds to those receptors. By doing so, it does not increase production of endometrial cells, nor does it change the makeup of vaginal cells. Also, it does not exert estrogen-like effects on the endometrium or breast, nor does it exhibit any toxic, mutagenic, or carcinogenic properties.

Given its apparent safety, I consider black cohosh a safe therapy for women who suffer from the acute symptoms of menopause, such as hot flashes, night sweats, sleeplessness, vaginal dryness and mood swings. Klimadynon from BioNorica has been shown to be an excellent source of black cohosh. Compelling research from several different journals, including *Maturitas: The European Menopause Journal* and *Menopause: The Journal of the North American Menopause Society*, has shown that Klimadynon (CR BNO 1055) safely and effectively eases hot flashes and night sweats, promotes plumping of the vaginal wall, decreases vaginal dryness, and even promoted bone growth. Moreover, Klimadynon did not cause proliferation of the uterine lining or of breast cells. This means that it, very likely, does not increase your risk of uterine or breast cancer.

Note: A study from the *Australian Adverse Drug Reactions Bulletin* found that, in rare instances, black cohosh can cause liver toxicity. More common and minor effects include occasional gastrointestinal disturbances, headaches, heaviness in the legs, and possible weight problems. There are no known drug interactions and the only contraindication is in pregnancy, with the possibility of premature birth due to overdose.

Additionally, an article in the *Journal of Agricultural & Food Chemistry* found that some three of 11 tested black cohosh supplements didn't even contain the herb! Instead, they contained less expensive extracts of a similar Chinese herb. To be sure this doesn't happen to you, I suggest buying black cohosh from a reputable retailer or look for BioNorica's Klimadynon brand.

To treat your menopausal symptoms safely and effectively, **I suggest taking 40–80 mg of a standardized extract of black cohosh such as Klim-adynon twice a day. This dose should contain 2 to 4 mg of the active components (triterpenes, calculated as 27-deoxyacteine).** You should see results within four weeks. In my practice, I have seen women experience relief from hot flashes and mood swings in as little as two days to one week.

Jennifer's Story

Jennifer called me in a panic and said that she needed to come in and see me right away. Her menopause symptoms were making her feel so nervous and stressed that she felt shaky all the time, was unable to sleep because of her hot flashes or even concentrate well. She was on constant deadlines with her job and was terrified that she would be fired because she was having difficulty completing her assignments. As a single woman who was helping to support her own mother who was ill and bedridden, she could not afford to lose her income.

When I saw Jennifer, she was distraught and obviously very worried. She was an attractive and nicely dressed woman but appeared pale and shaken. She did not want to take conventional HRT since she had had very uncomfortable side effects with oral contraceptives years earlier that made her feel bloated and anxious. She was concerned that conventional HRT would aggravate her current symptoms.

I felt that Jennifer was an excellent candidate for black cohosh and recommended that she try this as an option, along with a high quality multi-nutrient supplement, additional vitamin E, vitamin C and bioflavonoids. I also recommended that she avoid all coffee, sugar and alcohol, which could aggravate he nervousness, shakiness and hot flashes. She began the program immediately. I received a phone call from her within a few days, telling me that she was feeling much better, more calm and grounded and was able to work more effectively.

Red Clover

Red clover can also be useful for easing hot flashes and improving cardiovascular health. Red clover contains four phytoestrogens (estrogen-like plant compounds thought to have an effect on menopause-related symptoms such as hot flashes) called genistein, daidzein, biochanin, and formononetin, and has become increasingly popular among menopausal women here in the United States.

While some studies have questioned the efficacy of red clover, comparing it to that of a placebo, it does appear to help reduce hot flashes. According to a review of five studies published in *The American Journal of Medicine*, red clover helps to significantly reduce the frequency of hot flashes. Other research has shown that the herb is also beneficial for cardiovascular health. Both the aging process and menopause itself reduce the elasticity of major arteries (called arterial compliance). This tends to make blood vessels more rigid and less flexible. Over time, these changes can lead to high blood pressure, or hypertension, and increase the workload on the heart. In one placebo-controlled study reported in the *Journal of Clinical Endocrinology and Metabolism*, red clover improved arterial compliance. Other known potential cardiovascular benefits of red clover isoflavones include the inhibition of platelet clumping or aggregation, which can clog arteries, and the herb's action as a potent antioxidant, which also helps reduce buildup of "bad" LDL cholesterol in arteries. **I recommend taking a standardized extract that contains 40 mg of total isoflavones.**

Restoring the Yin

Traditional Asian medicine maintains that health and well-being are believed to be a balance of two equally important, but opposing, principles—yin and yang. Yin is associated with attributes such as femininity, receptivity, calmness, coolness, and moisture. Yin also regulates the fluids, blood, and tissues of your body, as well as its structural components, including flesh, tendons, and bones. Yang, on the other hand, is associated with masculinity, aggression, heat, and dryness. It also regulates your body's energy, which acts as the spark plug to your structural elements.

Balance between yin and yang is essential if you are to achieve and maintain optimal health and well-being. In younger, healthy women, the balance between this duality seems to be maintained almost effortlessly. Young women can become either very yin or very yang in response to the demands and stresses in their lives. They can study hard, work overtime, eat anything they want, and still have the ability to return to the balanced middle point, where yin and yang co-exist as a unified reality.

Maintaining an optimal yin-yang balance becomes much more difficult once you reach middle age and menopause, when it's common to experience symptoms such as hot flashes, night sweats, tissue dryness, insomnia, mood swings, and thinning of skin, hair, bones, and connective tissue. In the traditional Asian medical model, these symptoms occur, in part, because yin becomes deficient. To help bring your body back into balance, I suggest using a variety of yin herbs that work on the kidney network to improve blood and fluid circulation, ovarian health, and your sleep-wake cycle. In particular, I would like to focus on royal jelly, dong quai, saffron, rosewater and geranium oil.

Royal Jelly

Royal jelly—the food of the queen bee—has been used for centuries to promote reproductive health and longevity and ease menopausal symptoms. Doctors from France have reported that women who ate royal jelly during menopause had a complete remission of symptoms, and some were even able to conceive again! Other doctors have found that royal jelly had a libido-increasing effect and helped promote vaginal secretions. Additionally, royal jelly has been found to be a natural antibiotic, fat metabolizer, immune booster, and metabolic catalyst, and even supports adrenal health. I recommend using **1/4 teaspoon of the liquid form of organic royal jelly twice a day**.

Additionally, women who are allergic to bees or have asthma should not take royal jelly. Be sure to avoid royal jelly from China. Recent reports have shown that royal jelly imported from this country has been found to contain trace amounts of a dangerous antibiotic called chloramphenicol. To avoid this concern, be sure to purchase royal jelly that is produced by bees from the United States under healthy, organic conditions. Royal jell can be purchased at most health food stores or ordered from Glory Bee at glorybee.com or 800-456-7923. I like the Glory Bee products for my own personal use and have been using their products for many years!

Dong Quai

Dong quai is a Chinese herb (also called dang gui) that has been used for thousands of years as a female health tonic and to prevent or treat symptoms of PMS and menopause. Traditionally, dong quai has been used to treat abnormal menstruation and menopausal hot flashes. Many naturopathic physicians and herbalists today regularly prescribe this herb for their female patients.

In China, most women consume dong quai as a food, cooking the root in soup or other liquid mixture to soften it. **I recommend that you take dong quai in powdered form in a 500 mg capsule. Take two capsules two to three times a day.** Do not take dong quai if you are on a blood-thinner, as it may reinforce the effect of the anticoagulants and could increase your risk for bleeding.

Saffron

Saffron is a bright yellow Indian spice that is also used traditionally to reduce menopausal symptoms, enhance calmness, and reduce irritability. To preserve its medicinal properties, stir saffron into hot, cooked food. **Use 1/10 of a teaspoon or less per day, as higher amounts can be toxic**, causing stomach and intestinal maladies. Additionally, too much saffron can have a narcotic effect, causing sedation and sleepiness.

Formula D-34

I also want to tell you about an amazing multi-herb blend called **Formula D-34**. This impressive blend of 10 herbs also works to restore kidney yin. In fact, a study of 20 menopausal women found that Formula D-34 significantly increased blood levels of estradiol, the most potent and chemically active estrogen produced by your body. Additionally, the women reported a considerable reduction in menopausal symptoms, including hot flashes, depression, and anxiety. Formula D-34 is made by Draco Natural Products. I have included this amazing formula as one of the components in my own hormonal support product that I formulated for women with estrogen deficiency.

Rosewater

Water infused with rose oil supports the yin and has a calming and cooling effect on the body. It is an excellent topical to **spray on the skin several times a day** if you are experiencing heat symptoms such as hot flashes, dry skin and hair, wrinkling, restless sleep, and insomnia. It helps to hydrate the skin and is gentle and non-irritating. It also acts as an anti-inflammatory and is soothing to irritated skin. Rosewater has a delightful, sweet scent.

Geranium Oil

This essential oil has a lovely, feminine scent and blends well with other essential oils. It supports the yin, which is very helpful for women in menopause, and has a calming, harmonizing effect on the mood and emotions. Many women describe its effect as relaxing and uplifting. It can be used by women of all ages, but is particularly helpful for women in menopause. **Geranium essential oil can be added to bath water and is often incorporated into skin care products.** It benefits the dry skin that affects many women in menopause and has also been used for inflammatory conditions like acne and eczema.

Vitamins that Reduce Menopause Symptoms

Like phytoestrogens found in plants and herbs, certain vitamins have also been found to offer a natural way to reduce the symptoms of menopause—such as hot flashes, night sweats, insomnia, headaches, nervousness, and irritability—with little risk of side effects. The two vitamins with the most research in the area of menopause are and bioflavonoids.

Vitamin E

The original research on vitamin E's usefulness as an estrogen substitute was done between the 1930s and the early 1950s. Some of this research was done on breast and uterine cancer patients who were in menopause and were known to be poor candidates for estrogen replacement therapy, since it was understood as far back as the 1930's and 1940's that estrogen could stimulate the growth of any remaining tumor cells. Vitamin E was found to be both effective and safe in alleviating menopausal symptoms in these patients, and it could be safely used by breast cancer patients. Between 67 and 95 percent of the women followed in various studies had relief of such common menopausal symptoms as hot flashes, fatigue, mood swings, and muscle aches and pains. Vitamin E was less successful for the treatment of vaginal atrophy, being helpful in only 50 percent of the cases.

One such study from the *British Medical Journal* found that vitamin E not only helped reduce hot flashes in 64 percent of women tested, but also helped reduce symptoms of vaginal aging. Fifty percent of the women reported healing of vaginal atrophy, as well as a decrease in pain during sex.

A similar study published in the *Journal of the American Medical Association* found that of the 25 menopausal women treated with 10 mg of vitamin E, all found either complete relief or significant improvement in frequency and severity of hot flashes, as well as an improved mood and outlook on life. In another study of 66 women with menopause-related depression and irritability, 91 percent of the women found relief from their symptoms with vitamin E.

To relieve menopause-related symptoms, I suggest you take 400–1600 IU of natural vitamin E daily, as d-alpha in a base of mixed tocopherols. Start with a lower dose and increase this by 400 IU every two weeks until the desired effect is achieved.

Oil-based capsules can also be used topically to treat irritation caused by the thinning of the vaginal walls that can occur at menopause. The capsule is opened and the vitamin oil applied directly to vaginal tissues. I recommend that women test the vitamin first to make sure that there is no skin reaction. A tiny amount of vitamin E can be applied over a few days before using larger doses topically.

Bioflavonoids

These substances are found in the peel and pulp of citrus fruits as well as in buckwheat. While bioflavonoids can be useful in helping relieve and prevent premenopausal symptoms, they can be equally useful for menopausal women. This is because bioflavonoids are a subclass of flavonoids called flavones, which are weakly estrogenic. Happily, they can be used as a safe, nontoxic substitute for estrogen.

The potency of bioflavonoids is so low that they have no side effects for most women, yet they can relieve hot flashes as well as vaginal dryness. A study of ninety-four women at Loyola University Medical School showed the effectiveness of a bioflavonoids–vitamin C combination in controlling hot flashes for most of the women tested. In addition, bioflavonoids were used in this particular study as an estrogen substitute for cancer patients who cannot use traditional replacement therapy because their tumors are estrogen-sensitive. **I suggest taking 750–2,000 mg of bioflavonoids per day.** Bioflavonoids are considered to be very safe and have virtually no side effects.

Marla's Story

When Marla came to see me, she was 37 years old and had already had a total hysterectomy as a result of endometriosis. Her case of endometriosis had been quite severe, with years of ever-worsening menstrual cramps, which began 10 to 12 days before each menstrual cycle. She also experienced pain during the middle of her cycle, around the time of ovulation.

Marla also had endometrial implants in her colon, which caused painful bowel movements and intestinal irritability, as well as an irritable bladder. Unfortunately, the hysterectomy only swapped her problems for a set of new ones. Thanks to her "surgical menopause" she now had severe hot flashes, vaginal dryness, and sleeplessness, as well as extreme fatigue.

Her physician prescribed conventional hormone replacement therapy, which she could not tolerate due to the fact that it reactivated her endometriosis! Marla was very depressed and upset when she finally came to see me. She said that she literally felt trapped with no place to turn.

Luckily, my hormonal support and balancing program, including bioflavonoids, vitamin E, flaxseed and a number of other supportive nutrients and therapies like acupuncture proved to be very helpful, and her symptoms started to resolve.

15

Support Your Own Estrogen Production

You can also support hormone production in the central nervous system, ovaries, and adrenal glands, as well as reduce the breakdown and elimination of estrogen safely and gently with the use of specific nutrients. These can be used instead of or in addition to the hormone substitutes that I discussed in the previous chapter.

Because all hormone production begins in the brain, you can work to increase estrogen production through the brain or central nervous system. The hypothalamus is the master endocrine gland contained within your brain that regulates your production of sex hormones. This gland produces precursor hormones called gonadotropin releasing hormones (GnRH). When they are released, they travel to your anterior pituitary gland, where they stimulate the secretion of the follicle stimulating (FSH) and luteinizing hormones (LH). As you now know, these hormones then travel to the adrenals and ovaries, where they stimulate the production of estrogen, progesterone, and testosterone.

In order to keep the whole process working smoothly, FSH and LH need to be triggered by a balanced mixture of the key neurotransmitters necessary to produce these hormones. Neurotransmitters are naturally occurring chemicals that relay electrical messages between nerve cells throughout your body. The production of these vital chemicals is synthesized from certain amino acids, vitamins, and minerals that must be obtained through your diet or from supplementation.

For women who are in premenopause and are estrogen dominant, it is critical to increase levels of LH to help trigger ovulation and progesterone production. In the case of menopause and estrogen deficiency, just the opposite is true. You want to favor estrogen production. Additionally, you'll want to increase the neurotransmitter serotonin.

Serotonin: The Neurotransmitter for Peace and Calm

All neurotransmitters stimulate hormone production, but particularly menopausal women are most in need of serotonin. Serotonin is an inhibitory neurotransmitter. This means it quiets down the processes of your body, rather than speeding them up. Within your brain, serotonin often inhibits the firing of neurons, which dampens many of your behaviors. In fact, serotonin acts as a kind of chemical restraint system.

Of all your body's chemicals, serotonin has one of the most widespread effects on the brain and physiology. It plays a key role in regulating temperature, blood pressure, blood clotting, immunity, pain, digestion, sleep, and biorhythms. It also produces a relaxing effect on your mood.

When you are low in serotonin, you are most likely not a lot of fun to be around. Low levels often lead to mood swings, depression, insomnia, chronic pain, food cravings, migraine headaches, and irritable bowel syndrome. It can even increase your likelihood of infection and sleep apnea.

Menopausal women are most at risk of decreased levels of serotonin, thanks to a complementary relationship between this neurotransmitter and estrogen. According to research from both the *American Journal of Psychiatry* and *Behavioral and Cognitive Neuroscience Reviews*, as goes estrogen, so goes serotonin. It appears that estrogen stimulates serotonin production. If you don't have adequate amounts of estrogen, you are not producing adequate amounts of serotonin. Additionally, low estrogen also triggers your brain to release monoamine oxidase (MAO), an enzyme that degrades serotonin. So decreased estrogen levels have a double-whammy effect on serotonin.

This relationship is the key to postmenopausal depression and anxiety. By increasing estrogen, you increase serotonin, and thereby elevate your mood and reduce many of the symptoms related to menopause.

The essential amino acid tryptophan is initially converted into an inter-mediary substance called 5-hydroxytryptophan (5-HTP), which is then converted into serotonin. While tryptophan is available as a supplement and is abundant in turkey, pumpkin seeds, and almonds, I've found that 5-HTP is a more effective and reliable option for boosting your neurotransmitter production. Numerous double-blind studies have shown that 5-HTP is as effective as many of the more common antidepressant drugs and is associated with fewer and much milder side effects. In addition to increasing serotonin levels, 5-HTP triggers an increase in endorphins and other neurotransmitters that are often low in cases of depression.

The Serotonin-Thyroid Connection

Serotonin is also intimately bound with thyroid hormone. Healthy thyroid function plays an important role in supporting healthy serotonin production and concentration, as well as preventing serotonin reuptake. As a result, strong, healthy thyroid levels result in an increased level of serotonin in the brain.

If you exhibit symptoms of low thyroid—cold hands and/or feet, weight gain, constipation, fatigue, dry skin, brittle nails, depression, loss of hair—then you need to have a thyroid test performed. If you are determined to have low or hypothyroid, I strongly suggest bringing your thyroid hormone up to normal levels to ensure that you have adequate, healthy levels of serotonin.

To maintain proper serotonin levels, it is helpful to take 100–200 mg of 5-HTP per day, preferably at bedtime. I recommend with all nutritional supplements, you should start at the lower to more moderate dosage (100 mg a day). Stay on this dosage for two weeks. If you don't notice a reduction in your symptoms, gradually increase the dosage by 50 mg every two weeks until you have either noticed a reduction in your symptoms or have reached the maximum dosage.

Serotonin also needs to be properly balanced with other neurotransmitters that have a more excitatory effect on the body and stimulate energy, zest for life, libido and a more rapid metabolism. If you naturally have a more placid, peaceful temperament and a tendency towards lower energy, weight gain, fluid retention, and even depression, stimulating the brain's excitatory pathways that help to speed up the processes of your body will be more helpful for you.

The excitatory neurotransmitter pathways are primarily made up of substances like dopamine, norepinephrine, and epinephrine. Unlike serotonin, which has a calming and relaxing effect on your energy and behavior, excitatory neurotransmitters energize and elevate your mood. They act as powerful antidepressants and also support alertness, optimism, motivation, zest for life, and sex drive.

The excitatory neurotransmitters are derived from tyrosine, an amino acid produced from phenylalanine (another amino acid). A variety of vitamins and minerals, such as vitamin C, vitamin B6, and magnesium, act as cofactors and are necessary for the conversion of these amino acids into neurotransmitters.

To maintain optimum dopamine levels, take 500-1,000 mg of tyrosine per day. Be sure to take in divided doses, half in the morning and half in the afternoon. Do not take in the evening, as it may interfere with sleep.

Because creating a proper healthy balance between these two groups of neurotransmitters can be more challenging, I strongly advise that you undertake a program to properly balance your neurotransmitter levels under the care of a complementary physician or naturopath.

You should also have your neurotransmitter levels tested regularly. State-of-the-art neurotransmitter testing is currently available and can accurately pinpoint your exact levels of these essential brain chemicals. NeuroScience, Inc., (888-342-7272 or neurorelief.com) is a leader in the development of neurotransmitter testing. They have developed sensitive testing for these neurochemicals that can be done through your urine. The test is simple to do, non-invasive, and can be done in the privacy of your own home. In addition to NeuroScience, there are many other similar laboratories that offer neurotransmitter testing.

I would strongly recommend that you consider such testing if you suspect that you suffer from a moderate to severe neurotransmitter deficiency. Your health care provider will need to order these tests for you.

There are three key nutrients that will also help to raise estrogen levels—melatonin, glandulars, and ginseng through their effect on the brain and endocrine system. Let's take a look at each of them in more detail.

Melatonin

Melatonin is a hormone produced from serotonin and secreted by the pineal gland. Its secretion takes place at night and is inhibited by light. As such, it sets and regulates the timing of your body's natural circadian rhythms, such as waking and sleeping.

Unfortunately, as you get older, you produce less and less melatonin. This is due, in part, to menopause. Women how have poor sleep patterns, such as night shift workers, are also more likely to have decreased melatonin production.

As I mentioned earlier, melatonin is produced from serotonin, and serotonin production is stimulated by estrogen. Low estrogen equates to low serotonin, which results in low melatonin -- which means you can't fall asleep or stay asleep easily.

In fact, a study from the *Annals of the New York Academy of Sciences* found that there is a cause-effect relationship between decreased nighttime levels of melatonin and the onset of menopause. Researchers found that women who took 3 mg of melatonin a day for six months enjoyed decreased FSH levels (with levels returning to those of a younger woman), and nearly a third of the menopausal women experienced a return of normal menstrual cycles. Even though estrogen and other hormone levels were not elevated during the study, a return of menstruation means more estrogen production. And, as I mentioned earlier, when women enter menopause, their levels of FSH and LH production in the pituitary increase in an effort to trigger greater estrogen production. Additionally, the study showed a significant improvement in thyroid function and relief of menopause-related depression in the women using melatonin.

Another research study published in the *Journal of Clinical Endocrinology and Metabolism* studied men and women over the age of 50 who suffered from insomnia to assess the best melatonin dosage necessary to promote healthy sleep. Researchers looked at three dosages: 0.1 mg; 0.3 mg; and 3.0 mg (the same dosage used in the *Annals of the New York Academy of Sciences* study). Unfortunately, they found that the 3.0 mg dosage had some downsides. It decreased body temperature and caused melatonin levels to stay elevated throughout the day. However, the lower doses—especially the 0.3 mg dosage—restored sleep without these negative side effects.

Research has also shown that melatonin is cancer-protective. One study looked at 250 patients with a wide variety of advanced, metastatic tumors, including lung cancer, breast cancer, gastrointestinal cancer, and head and neck cancer. None of the patients who received chemotherapy alone enjoyed a complete response, while six of the patients who received chemo and 20 mg of intravenous melatonin did, and another 36 patients achieved a partial response. Moreover, the one-year survival rate was significantly higher in the melatonin/chemo group (51 percent) than the chemo-alone group (23 percent). Researchers concluded that melatonin may be the secret weapon in the war on cancer.

To ensure that you have adequate levels of melatonin, I suggest supplementing with 0.3–1 mg at bedtime. Some women may find that they do better with a higher dosage. In this case, I suggest taking 1.5–3 mg. In my own hormone support product, I have erred on the side of caution and included 0.3 mg of melatonin. For melatonin to be effective, your bedroom should be dark, as light suppresses its release.

The following drugs deplete melatonin. If you are taking these drugs, be sure to supplement with adequate amounts of melatonin.

- Aspirin
- Ibuprofen
- Beta-blockers
- Calcium channel blockers
- Sleeping pills
- Tranquilizers

> **Carol's Story**
>
> Carol was a 68-year-old patient of mine who, for about 15 years after reaching menopause, experienced mild depression and mood swings. When she came to see me, her depression had worsened and sleeplessness had set in. Even more frustrating for her was that she felt sleepy and depressed during the day, but as soon as the sun went down, she became restless and couldn't sleep for more than three hours. This cycle of sleepiness and sleeplessness was beginning to affect her work and even her simple, everyday tasks—but even more upsetting, her marriage was starting to sour.
>
> Carol's situation is common in women who have neurotransmitter imbalances. Testing showed that Carol did indeed have a neurotransmitter imbalance—in particular, her serotonin levels were too low.
>
> I put Carol on a combination of melatonin, valerian root as well as other nutrients. Soon, she was feeling like her old self again and sleeping better than ever.

Glandulars

Glandular therapy involves the use of purified extracts from the secretory endocrine glands of animals. Most commonly, extracts are drawn from the thyroid and adrenal glands, as well as the thymus, pituitary, pancreas, and ovaries. Most extracts come from cows, with the exception of pancreatic glandular preparations usually drawn from sheep.

There are four common ways to extract glandulars. The first involves quick-freezing the material, washing it with a potent solvent to remove fatty tissues, distilling the solvent out, drying it, and then grinding it into a fine powder that is then encapsulated or pressed into tablets. The second mixes freshly crushed material with salt and water that also removes fatty tissues. It is then dried and ground into a fine powder to be placed in capsules or made into tablets.

In the third method, the glandular material is freeze-dried, then placed into a vacuum chamber to remove the water. It is then encapsulated. However, with this method, fatty tissues remain. The final method uses plant and animal enzymes to partially "digest" the material. It is then passed through a filter that separates out the fat-soluble molecules. The remaining material is then freeze-dried. This method seems to be quite effective. Due to the "pre-digestion," all biologically active substances remain intact and can be used therapeutically to support and restore your body's endocrine glands. Healthier endocrine glands are more likely to create healthier hormone production.

In the past, most experts believed that glandulars were not effective because the intestinal lining of a healthy person was impenetrable, and that proteins and large peptides could not breach its barrier. However, recent evidence has shown that large macromolecules can and do pass completely intact from the intestinal tract and into the bloodstream. In fact, there's further evidence to suggest that your body is able to determine which molecules it needs to absorb whole, and which can be broken down.

Both animal and human studies alike have proven this theory. In some cases, several whole proteins taken orally, including critical enzymes, have been shown to be absorbed intact into the bloodstream. Additionally, many smaller proteins and numerous hormones have also been found to be absorbed intact into the bloodstream, including thyroid, cortisone, and even insulin.

In essence, it means that the active properties of the glandulars stay active and intact, and are not destroyed in the digestive process. This is key to the success of glandular therapy, and explains why they clearly help to restore hormone function. When the gland is healthy, you de facto have fewer hormone-related problems because the feedback loop of the central nervous system and the endocrine glands are working properly. In essence, if you optimize the function, you bring *all* your hormones back into balance.

Examples of widely used and accepted glandulars involve the thyroid and the adrenals. Natural thyroid medications such as Armour Thyroid, Naturthyroid, and Bio-Thyroid have been the preference of complementary physicians for decades. Unlike many of the commonly prescribed brands of thyroid therapy that only replace a synthetic form of T4, these natural thyroid replacements contains the whole animal-derived thyroid gland, including T3 *and* T4. This is a significant difference. T3 is more physiologically active than T4, and is critical in regulating normal growth and energy metabolism. Without the use of glandulars, this type of natural thyroid replacement wouldn't be possible. However, the thyroid glandulars sold in the health food stores have the hormone removed and are used to support the function of your own gland.

Adrenal glandular preparations are even more common. With the stress epidemic in this country, the majority of Americans are walking around with major adrenal stress. Fortunately, whole adrenal extracts have been found to help restore the health and function of comprised adrenal glands. In one research study, eight women suffering from morning sickness (nausea and vomiting) who took oral adrenal cortex extract found relief within four days. A similar study gave both injected and oral adrenal cortex extract to 202 women also suffering from morning sickness. More than 85 percent of the women completely overcame their nausea and vomiting or showed significant improvement.

To support the endocrine glands that make estrogen (and other female hormones), as well as those that regulate estrogen production—including the pineal gland, which secretes melatonin—I suggest taking a good multi-glandular or single glandular product such as pineal or hypothalamus from a company like Standard Process. Standard Process is a leader in the field; however, they do require a prescription from a health care practitioner. Other good products are also available in health food stores and should be used as part of a nutritional program to support your entire hormone system. I suggest consulting with a complementary health care provider if you are interested in using glandular therapy.

Ginseng

Panax ginseng is an ivy-like ground cover originating in the wild, damp woodlands of northern China and Korea. Its use in Chinese herbal medicine dates back more than 4,000 years. In colonial North America, ginseng was a major export product. The wild form is now rare, but panax ginseng is a widely cultivated plant.

Ginseng has a legendary status among herbs. While extravagant claims have been made about its many uses, scientific research has yielded inconsistent results in verifying its therapeutic properties. However, enough good research does exist to demonstrate ginseng's activity, especially when high-quality extracts, standardized for active components, are used.

Ginseng has a balancing, tonic effect on the systems and organs of the body involved in the stress response. It contains at least 13 different saponins, a class of chemicals found in many plants, especially legumes, which take their name from their ability to form a soap-like froth when shaken with water. These compounds (triterpene glycosides) are the most pharmaceutically active constituents of ginseng. Saponins benefit cardiovascular function, hormone production, immunity, and the central nervous system.

During times of stress, ginseng acts as a general stimulant, delaying the alarm phase in Selye's classic model of stress. The saponins in the ginseng act on the hypothalamus and pituitary glands, increasing the release of adrenocorticotrophin, or ACTH (a hormone produced by the pituitary that promotes the manufacture and secretion of adrenal hormones). As a result, ginseng increases the release of adrenal cortisone and other adrenal hormones, including estrogen, and prevents their depletion from stress. Other substances associated with the pituitary are also released, such as endorphins.

In a double-blind study published in *Drugs Under Experimental and Clinical Research*, two groups of volunteers suffering from fatigue due to physical or mental stress were given nutritional supplementation over a 12-week period. One hundred sixty-three volunteers were given a multivitamin and multi-mineral complex, and 338 volunteers received the same product plus a standardized Chinese ginseng extract. Once a month, the volunteers were asked to fill out a questionnaire during a scheduled visit with a physician. This questionnaire contained 11 questions that asked them to describe their current level of perceived physical energy, stamina, sense of well-being, libido, and quality of sleep.

While both groups experienced similar improvement in their quality of life by the second visit, the group using the ginseng extract almost doubled their improvement, based on their questionnaire responses, by the third and fourth visits. Thus, ginseng, when added to a multivitamin and multi-mineral complex, appears to improve many parameters of well-being in individuals experiencing significant physical and emotional stress. This is particularly important for women in menopause with diminished estrogen production.

Ginseng also enhances mental capacity, as demonstrated in both animal studies and clinical trials in humans. Improvements in logical deduction, reaction time, mental arithmetic, alertness, and accuracy have been observed. ACTH (the hormone that stimulates the adrenal cortex) and adrenal hormones, which ginseng stimulates, are known to bind to brain tissue, increasing mental activity and acuity during stress.

Many of my patients have used ginseng and have found it to have energizing effects. When trying to replace yin, I suggest using the more cooling Chinese and American forms of ginseng, and avoid Korean red ginseng, which is considered to be "hotter" and more yang. This type of ginseng can have the reverse effect, causing a decrease in normal menstrual flow and dryness of the skin and mucous membranes.

To further support hormone function at the central nervous system level, I suggest taking 100 mg of American or Chinese ginseng in capsule form twice a day. For maximum benefit, be sure to take a high-quality preparation, standardized for ginsenoside content and ratio. If this is too stimulating, especially before bedtime, take the second dose mid-afternoon, or take only the morning dose.

In addition to stimulating hormone production at the endocrine and nervous system levels, you can also use nutrients such as wheat germ oil and boron to increase estrogen production.

Nutrients that Increase Estrogen Production

Wheat Germ Oil

Wheat germ oil is rich in vitamin E, which we already know has mildly estrogenic properties. In fact, wheat germ oil contains the same fatty acids and other nutrients like vitamin E that your body needs to support and produce hormones such as estrogen.

Wheat germ oil is so effective, it has even been shown to increase estrogen production and reestablish healthy menstrual cycles in young women. Living under the stress of war is often associated with widespread disruption of menstrual cycles. This was true of women living in an internment camp in Manila during World War II. Doctors who treated these women observed that menstruation had stopped abruptly after the first bombing of Manila, before a nutritional deficiency would have been experienced. These physicians conducted a small study, published in the *Journal of the American Medical Association* (JAMA), in which 10 women with amenorrhea (a lack of menstruation) were given 20 drops of wheat germ oil as a source of vitamin E. The doses were taken orally, three times a day, for a period of 10 days, preceding the onset of each woman's expected menstrual flow. Of the 10 women, eight began to menstruate or had uterine bleeding.

Another study found that wheat germ oil was beneficial in treating vaginitis in menopausal women. One particular patient had such an extreme case of the condition that the physician couldn't even examine her. After 10 days on wheat germ oil, the burning eased and 17 days later, she reported to be "feeling better than she had in months".

I've found wheat germ oil to be very effective in treating the entire range of menopausal symptoms, most notably hot flashes. **I suggest taking 2,000–2,400 mg of wheat germ oil in capsule form a day, in divided doses.** I recommend Viobin and Standard Process brands (viobinusa.com and standardprocess.com).

Boron

Boron is a trace mineral found in foods such as apples, grapes, almonds, legumes, honey, and dark green leafy vegetables like kale and beet greens. According to a study conducted by the U.S. Department of Agriculture, there is some evidence that boron enhances estrogenic activity. When women on estrogen therapy supplemented their normally low-boron diet with 3 mg of boron, their blood levels of estrogen, specifically beta-estradiol, were significantly elevated. It appears that boron boosts estrogen production and mimics some effects of estrogen. There is also anecdotal evidence that boron may reduce hot flashes.

Moreover, boron is critical in the fight against osteoporosis. One study published in *Nutrition Today* found that boron reduced urinary excretion of calcium by 44 percent and significantly reduced excretion of magnesium as well. It also found that it increased levels of both beta-estradiol and testosterone. **To help boost estrogen levels and prevent osteoporosis, I suggest taking 3 mg of boron a day.**

Nutrients that Decrease the Breakdown and Elimination of Estrogen

While plant-based nutrients, vitamins, and minerals all work to support estrogen production, you can also decrease the metabolism and elimination of estrogen to help maintain higher levels of the hormone. This will also help to relieve symptoms of estrogen deficiency. Let's take a look at the best ways to accomplish this.

Women with estrogen dominance need to be sure they are breaking down, metabolizing, and eliminating excess estrogen effectively. However, women in estrogen deficiency need to do everything they can to slow down this breakdown and excretion cycle.

During estrogen metabolism in the liver, the most potent estrogen (estradiol) is converted into the mid-level potency form of estrone. They are both then metabolized to the weakest and least potent form — estriol.

Estrogen is also inactivated as it passes through the liver, where it is bound to sulfuric and glucuronic acid. This binding process inactivates the estrogen, inhibiting it from binding to tissues. It is then secreted into the bile and passed into the intestinal tract, where it is then eliminated from the body via bowel movements.

To slow this process down, you need hormone potentiators, nutrients that help to keep free estrogen from being reabsorbed by the body, thus elevating the level of estrogen circulating through the body. That's where PABA and cobalt chloride (or cobalt derived from vitamin B12) come in.

PABA

PABA (para-aminobenzoic acid) is a fat-soluble B vitamin necessary for the production of folic acid. It helps to break down protein in the body, support red blood cell production, and maintain the health of the intestines. PABA also works to absorb ultraviolet light, and may be useful in alleviating some skin conditions, such as the over-pigmentation or under-pigmentation of skin.

More importantly, studies indicate that PABA helps to safely and effectively impede the breakdown of estrogen and other hormones in the liver. Research has shown that higher levels of PABA are associated with better mood and outlook, less thinning hair, better vaginal lubrication, and increased libido — all of which are also indicative of higher estrogen levels. In fact, PABA is the only substance (other than testosterone) that has been proven to increase libido!

In addition to increasing estrogen levels, PABA has also been found to increase adrenal and thyroid hormone levels, as well as enhance the effects of cortisone. Because of its cortisone-like effects, PABA was used to treat rheumatoid arthritis in the 1940's. Specifically, PABA has been shown to be beneficial in helping to relieve the stiffness and pain associated with arthritis. In fact, high doses of PABA have been found to prevent and even reverse the accumulation of fibrous tissue.

One study from the *American Journal of Medical Sciences* found that rheumatoid arthritis sufferers who took a low doses of cortisone and high doses of PABA enjoyed considerable pain relief. Specifically, they found that patients who took 12 grams of PABA, along with low amounts of cortisone, enjoyed significantly more relief than those people taking cortisone alone.

Moreover, PABA has also been found to be effective in overcoming infertility. Researchers gave 16 infertile women 100 mg of PABA four times a day for three to seven months. Twelve of the 16 become pregnant.

If you are tired, depressed, irritable, or show signs of anxiety, you may be deficient in PABA. **I recommend taking 400 mg a day, which may be taken in divided dosages as a hormone potentiator. To reduce pain associated with arthritis, take 4–10 grams of PABA.**

Linda's Story

Linda was 71 years old when she first came to see me. She had been taking conventional HRT for nearly 20 years. When she read the study results published in the *Journal of the American Medical Association* on the connection between synthetic HRT and heart disease and breast cancer, she quit taking her medications cold turkey.

Within days, she began experiencing terrible hot flashes, worse than she remembered from her early 50's. She also had insomnia, which kept her up most nights. She started using PABA, glandulars, and a few other nutrients to help ease her symptoms. She was delighted to find that her symptoms decreased in a very short period of time.

Cobalt

One of the most exciting, and little known, nutrients for menopausal women is cobalt. Research has shown that cobalt slows down the excretion of estrogen, thus allowing you to better maintain own production of estrogen, as well as that of supplemental estrogen.

Cobalt is able to retain estrogen and other hormones by stimulating production of heme oxidase. This, in turn, promotes the breakdown of cytochrome p450, a substance that normally metabolizes and detoxifies estrogen. By breaking down this substance, cobalt helps to prevent estrogen metabolism and excretion.

Physicians who have used cobalt have found that it has significant therapeutic benefits for their patients, helping to reduce night sweats, insomnia, hot flashes, depression, mood swings, and memory loss. It has even improved the therapeutic effects of women using conventional HRT who were not experiencing symptom relief due to their hyperexcreting of the hormones.

To impede the breakdown and excretion of estrogen, I suggest taking 400–500 mcg of cobalt a day. To further improve your cobalt status, you can also take 100–500 mcg of B12 a day. Research has shown that cobalt is supplied in your body by B12. If you have adequate amounts of B12, you are likely to have adequate amounts of cobalt as well.

16

Vitamins, Minerals & Essential Fatty Acids for Specific Symptom Relief

In this chapter, I take a symptom relief approach for menopause. I discuss how specific vitamins, minerals, and fatty acids can help to relieve a wide variety of menopause symptoms. Since women vary greatly in the types and severity of symptoms that they experience with menopause, this chapter will be very useful in helping you to create a program customized to your own needs.

I have found nutritional supplementation to be very helpful in providing symptom relief to thousands of patients dealing with menopause related health issues. The important role nutritional supplements can play in helping reduce the symptoms of premenopause and menopause, as well as the risk of common postmenopausal health problems, is supported by many medical research studies done at university centers and hospitals (a bibliography is provided at the end of this book).

The use of supplements must go hand-in-hand with a low-stress, healthful diet. It is not enough to take supplements while continuing poor dietary habits. Women who try this do not achieve the results they're looking for. However, diet alone often cannot provide the nutrient levels necessary for the most complete relief of menopausal symptoms. Supplements can speed up and facilitate the return to optimal health and well-being.

This chapter is divided into two sections. In the first section, the role of vitamins, minerals and essential fatty acids in symptom relief and prevention is discussed. In the second section, I provide specific recommendations, usage tips, and optimal nutritional formulas for premenopausal and menopausal women. Also included are charts listing major food sources of each essential nutrient discussed.

Vitamins and Minerals for Relieving Specific Menopausal Symptoms

Heavy and Irregular Bleeding

Vitamin A. Heavy menstrual bleeding is a significant problem for premenopausal women due to the production of excessive amounts of estrogen or the accelerated growth of fibroids. Excessive bleeding is also one of the most common reasons for hysterectomies. Luckily, vitamin A can play a role in reducing these symptoms.

In a study of seventy-one women with excessive bleeding, the women had significantly lower blood levels of vitamin A than the average population. After two weeks of vitamin A treatment, almost 90 percent of the women studied returned to a normal bleeding pattern. Vitamin A promotes normal growth and support for the eyes, skin, mucous membranes, red blood cells and healthy immune function. Deficiency of vitamin A results in impaired immune function, rough, scaly skin and night blindness.

Vitamin A is found in two forms. Vitamin A from animal sources, usually from fish liver, is oil soluble. This type of vitamin A can be toxic if taken in too large a dose (greater than 25,000 international units [IU] per day for more than a few months). In contrast, beta carotene, the precursor of vitamin A found in plants, is water soluble and is not toxic in large amounts. A single sweet potato or cup of carrot juice contains more than 20,000 IU of beta carotene. **I recommend 5,000 to 20,000 IU per day taken as a supplement.**

Vitamin B Complex. Vitamin B complex consists of 11 factors that perform many important biochemical functions in the body. These include stabilization of brain chemistry, glucose metabolism and the inactivation of estrogen by the liver. Since heavy menstrual bleeding can be triggered by excess estrogen in the body, it is important that estrogen levels are properly regulated through breakdown and disposal by the liver. In pioneering animal and human research in 1942 and 1943, Morton S. Biskind highlighted the important role of several B-complex vitamins in regulating estrogen levels through promoting healthy liver function. Women with several problems related to excessive estrogen levels, inclu-ding heavy menstrual flow, PMS and fibrocystic breast disease received supplements of vitamin B complex. When supplemented with thiamine (B1), riboflavin (B2), niacin and niacinamide (B3), as well as the rest of the B complex, the women in this research study showed relief from estrogen-related symptoms.

In women with heavy menstrual bleeding, **I generally recommend 50 to 100 mg per day of vitamin B complex**. The B vitamins are water soluble and easily lost from the body. Emotional and nutritional stress accelerates the loss of these essential nutrients from the body. This can increase other symptoms seen with fibroids and endometriosis including fatigue, faint-ness and dizziness. Besides supplementation, a diet high in B complex is desirable for women. The B-complex vitamins are commonly found in food such as whole grains, beans, peas and liver.

Vitamin C. Vitamin C has been tested, along with bioflavonoids, as a treatment for heavy menstrual bleeding. One research project showed a reduction in bleeding in 87 percent of the women participating in the study. Dozens of similar studies showing the efficacy of vitamin C and bioflavonoids for the treatment of heavy bleeding. Vitamin C reduces bleeding by strengthening capillaries. Women who bleed excessively may eventually become iron deficient and develop anemia. Vitamin C increases iron absorption from food sources such as bran, peas, seeds, nuts, and leafy green vegetables, thus helping prevent iron-deficiency anemia.

I recommend that women with excessive bleeding use 1000 to 4000 mg of vitamin C per day, especially when symptoms occur. Many fruits and vegetables are excellent sources of vitamin C.

Bioflavonoids. Like vitamin C, substances called bioflavonoids, have shown dramatic ability to reduce heavy menstrual bleeding through stren-gthening the capillary walls. Bioflavonoids also interfere with the body's estrogen production. This may be helpful to menopausal women who suffer from the effects of elevated estrogen levels, such as heavy bleeding, fibroid tumors, and PMS symptoms. Studies have shown that a bioflavonoid and vitamin C combination can reduce heavy menstrual bleeding by as much as 50 percent. Bioflavonoids produce this menstrual-regulating effect through the following mechanism: within the ovaries, estrogen production occurs as a result of the conversion of the male hormone testosterone into the female hormone estrogen. This reaction only occurs with the help of an enzyme, called estogen synthetase, to which the testosterone must bind. Bioflavonoids disrupt this process by competing with the testosterone for the binding site, thereby interfering with estogen production.

I generally recommend 500 to 2000 mg bioflavonoids per day in women with premenopausal bleeding problems. Bioflavonoids are found in grape skins, cherries, blackberries and blueberries as well as being abundant in citrus fruits, especially in the pulp and the white rind. They are also found in other foods such as buckwheat.

Iron. Women who suffer from premenopausal heavy menstrual bleeding run the risk of developing iron deficiency, the main cause of anemia. Iron is an essential component of red blood cells, combining with protein and copper to make hemoglobin, the pigment of the red blood cells. Iron deficiency is common during all phases of a woman's life and is a frequent cause of fatigue and low-energy states. In fact, some medical studies have found that inadequate iron intake may cause excessive bleeding.

Women who suffer from heavy menstrual bleeding should have their red blood count checked to see if supplemental iron is necessary, in addition to a high-iron-content diet. Heme iron, the iron from meat sources such as liver, is much better absorbed and assimilated than nonheme iron, the iron from vegetarian sources. To be absorbed properly, nonheme iron must be taken with at least 75 mg of vitamin C.

Good food sources of iron include liver, blackstrap molasses, beans, peas, seeds, nuts, certain fruits and vegetables. **I recommend 18-25mg per day of an iron supplement.**

Hot Flashes, Night Sweats, Vaginal and Bladder Atrophy

Vitamin A. Vitamin A is necessary for the growth and support of the skin and mucous membranes. As a result, this nutrient is very important for the support of the vulvar, vaginal and urinary tissues. Lack of vitamin A is a risk factor for developing bladder or cervical cancer and can predispose a woman to skin conditions related to the aging process, such as vulvar leukoplakia and senile keratosis. Both of these conditions can precede the onset of skin cancer.

Vitamin A is best from the vegetable source, beta-carotene. This is because vitamin A from animal sources can produce toxic symptoms such as headaches and liver damage if taken in excessive doses for periods longer than several months. However, the provitamin A, beta-carotene, is extremely safe. For women with vaginal and bladder atrophy, **I generally recommend between 25,000 to 100,000 IU per day**. (25,000 IU is found in one sweet potato or one cup of carrot juice.)

Vitamin C. Adequate amounts of vitamin C are needed to maintain the skin, including the vulvar, vaginal and bladder tissues. Vitamin C is necessary for collagen synthesis and skin strength. A low vitamin C intake has been found to predispose women to cervical dysplasia and cancer of the cervix.

The diet of women with early-stage cervical cancer has been compared to those of healthy controls in research studies. Women with cervical cancer were found to have a diet much lower in foods containing vitamin C. While vitamin C alone will not reverse bladder and vaginal atrophy, sufficient daily intake of this nutrient is necessary, along with vitamin A, to support these tissues.

I generally recommend between 1000 to 5000 mg per day for menopausal women. Side effects are rare, although some women find that higher doses cause diarrhea; if this happens to you, reduce the dose to a comfortable level. Rarely, large doses of vitamin C can predispose to kidney stones. Many fruits and vegetables as well as some meats contain high levels of vitamin C.

Isoflavones. The phytoestrogens found in soy have been shown to reduce hot flashes in studies comparing European or Canadian women with Asian women, for whom soy is an important part of their diet. A study, published in the *British Medical Journal*, also found soy to be useful in reducing vaginal atrophy. **Soy isoflavones can be ingested in premeasured doses of 40 to 60 mg in both capsules and powders, and are available in health food stores as well as a diet that is rich in soy-based foods.**

Bioflavonoids. A study of 94 women at Loyola University Medical School found a bioflavonoids-vitamin C combination to be helpful in controlling hot flashes. This study used a bioflavonoid called hesperidin in a dosage of 1200 mg per day, as well as 1200 mg per day of vitamin C. The study also concluded that bioflavonoids could be useful as an estrogen substitute for breast and uterine cancer patients who cannot use traditional hormone replacement therapy. Because of their blood vessel strengthening effect, bioflavonoids can help to reduce bruising and bleeding of the gums in menopausal women.

In my own practice **I usually recommend dosages of bioflavonoids varying from 500 to 2000 mg daily**. In more than two decades of clinical practice, I have rarely seen any adverse side effects from the use of bioflavonoids.

Vitamin E. Vitamin E has shown promise in research studies as a treatment for the most common menopausal symptoms, including hot flashes, night sweats, and even vaginal dryness. Depending on the study, between 66 to 85 percent of the women tested found vitamin E to be an effective substitute for estrogen. Vitamin E can be a useful treatment option for women who cannot, or do not, choose to use the higher potencies of prescription hormones. For example, one early research study in *The American Journal of Obstetrics and Gynecology* reported that nearly all 25 cancer patients they studied had an excellent response to vitamin E therapy. These women had become menopausal either through surgery or reduced dosage of hormone replacement. All had severe hot flashes and mood alterations that could not be treated by estrogen replacement therapy due to their types of tumors. Using vitamin E as an estrogen substitute, 23 out of the 25 women had either complete relief or significant improvement of their symptoms.

Another interesting study of 47 menopausal women reported in the *British Medical Journal* found that vitamin E not only helped reduce hot flashes in 64 percent of women tested, but also helped reduce symptoms of vaginal aging. Fifty percent of the women noted healing of vaginal atrophy as well as a decrease in pain during sexual intercourse. To repeat for emphasis, many women with vaginal atrophy are also prone to recurrent vaginal infections, which produce uncomfortable symptoms such as itching, burning and discharge. A study in *The American Journal of Obstetrics and Gynecology* reported that 44 women at high risk for developing yeast vaginitis because of a pre-existing diabetic condition noted significant relief of symptoms when treated with vitamin E vaginal suppositories.

Generally, I recommend using 400 to 1600 IU of vitamin E per day. Begin at a low dose and gradually increase the dosage over several weeks until you achieve the desired relief. Women with hypertension, diabetes or bleeding problems, however, should begin at much lower dosages of vitamin E (100 IU per day). If you have any of these conditions, ask your physician about the advisability of using vitamin E. In general, however, vitamin E tends to be well tolerated and is used by millions of people without adverse effects. Many women with severe vaginal atrophy use vitamin E topically. Besides taking vitamin E by mouth, you might try opening a capsule and applying the oil directly to your vaginal tissues. Vitamin E occurs abundantly in vegetable oils, raw nuts, seeds and in some fruits and vegetables.

Essential Fatty Acids. Essential fatty acids are particularly important to menopausal women because the deficiency of these oils is responsible, in part, for the drying of the vaginal and bladder mucosa as well as the skin, hair, and other tissues of the body that occur at midlife. The deficiency is primarily nutritional because these fats cannot be made by the body and must be supplied daily in your diet. The main sources of essential fatty acids are raw seeds and nuts or fish, which are not a usual part of the typical American diet.

Both whole ground flaxseeds, which are 50 percent oil by content, or purified oil in capsule form are excellent sources of the two essential oils, linoleic acid and alpha-linolenic acid. Flax meal was the oil source used in the study of vaginal atrophy reported in the *British Medical Journal*, though many women prefer to take essential fatty acids in capsule form. Fish oil taken as a supplement also provides essential omega 3 fatty acids, which reduce inflammation and support the health of the brain and heart. I recommend fish oil capsules containing a combination of 2000 to 3000 mg of EPA (eicosapentaenoic acid) and DHA (docosahexaenoic acid). Women who like the buttery taste of raw flax oil may want to take one to three tablespoons orally per day of flax oil.

Menopause-Related Emotional Symptoms and Insomnia

Vitamin B complex. The B vitamins play an important role in healthy nervous system function. When one or more of these vitamins are deficient, symptoms of nerve impairment, anxiety, stress and fatigue can result. Conversely, eating appropriate food sources and taking supplements of B vitamins can help calm the mood and provide important factors for a stable and constant source of energy. This can be very important during menopause when women's moods tend to fluctuate due to hormonal instability.

Consistent high levels of emotional stress trigger the fight-or-flight alarm response, which results in excessive output of adrenal hormones. Deficiencies of individual B vitamins also increase nervous tension and stress. Pantothenic acid (vitamin B5) is needed for healthy adrenal function. Pyridoxine (vitamin B6) also affects mood because it has an important role in the conversion of linoleic acid to gamma-linolenic acid (GLA) in the production of the beneficial series-one prostaglandins. Prostaglandins have a relaxant effect on both mood and smooth muscle tissue. Lack of these relaxant hormones has been linked to stress-related problems such as irritable bowel syndrome and migraine headaches.

Vitamin B6 levels may decrease in menopausal women who are using estrogen replacement therapy. (This can also be a problem for women using oral contraceptives, a common treatment for PMS, menstrual cramps and irregularity.) Anxiety symptoms can occur as a side effect of hormone use in both groups of women, in part because of B6 deficiency. **Vitamin B6 can be safely used in doses up to 150 mg; doses above this level should be avoided or used under a physician's care.**

Lack of B6 may also increase anxiety symptoms directly through its effect on the nervous system. The body needs B6 in order to convert the amino acid tryptophan to serotonin, an important neurotransmitter. Serotonin regulates sleep; when it is deficient, insomnia occurs. Sleeplessness is a condition menopausal women frequently suffer. Serotonin levels also strongly affect mood and social behavior. Both B6 and food sources of tryptophan such as almonds, pumpkin seeds, sesame seeds and certain other protein containing foods, are necessary for adequate serotonin production.

For women who fall asleep easily but can't return to sleep after awakening in the middle of the night, niacin (vitamin B3) may be helpful. Research studies have shown that niacinamide, a form of niacin, has effects similar to those in minor tranquilizers. In addition, inositol, another B vitamin, has been shown to have calming effects. Its effect on brain waves studied by electroencephalograph (EEG) were similar to changes induced by minor tranquilizers.

In summary, the entire range of B vitamins is needed in order to provide nutritional support to avoid anxiety and stress symptoms. Because B vitamins are water soluble, the body cannot readily store them. Thus, B vitamins must be consumed daily through diet. Good sources of most B vitamins include brewer's yeast (which many women cannot easily digest), liver, wheat germ and bran, beans, peas and nuts. Vitamin B12 is found primarily in animal foods. Women following a vegan diet (a vegetarian diet utilizing no dairy products or eggs) should take particular care to add supplemental vitamin B12 to their diets. **I recommend 25 to 100 mg of vitamin B-complex per day.**

Vitamin C. Vitamin C is an extremely important anti-stress nutrient that can help decrease the fatigue symptoms that often accompany excessive levels of nervous tension and stress. It is needed for the production of adrenal gland hormones. Activation of the fight-or-flight pattern in response to stress depletes these hormones. Larger amounts of vitamin C in the diet are needed when stress levels are high. In one research study done on 411 dentists and their spouses, scientists found a clear relationship between lack of vitamin C and the presence of fatigue.

The best sources of vitamin C in nature are fruits and vegetables. It is a water-soluble vitamin, so it is not stored in the body. Thus, menopausal women with anxiety and excessive stress should replenish their vitamin C supply daily through a healthy diet and the use of supplements. **I recommend 1000 to 3000 mg per day of mineral buffered vitamin C, taken in divided doses.**

Isoflavones. Isoflavones derived from soy beans have the property of being weakly estrogenic, which is helpful for the stress due to menopause-related hormonal deficiency. Since estrogen has a stimulant effect on the brain, the weakly estrogenic activity of the isoflavones can act as a mild mood elevator in hormonally deficient women. In nature, isoflavones are commonly found in soy foods. They are currently available in purified forms as powders, capsules, and bars. **Optimal dosages may be from 50 to 60 mg.**

Vitamin E. Like isoflavones, vitamin E relieves symptoms of anxiety and mood swings in women suffering from either menopause or PMS. In studies of vitamin E as an alternative treatment for menopause, it has relieved mood swings and reduced other menopause-related symptoms. For example in one study of 66 women with menopause-related depression, tearfulness and irritability, as well as hot flashes, 60 women found that to vitamin E, relieved their emotional symptoms. Some women find that conventional estrogen therapy increases their anxiety symptoms. These women are potentially good candidates for vitamin E therapy.

I generally recommend that women with menopause-related anxiety and mood swings use between 400 to 1600 IU per day. Women with hypertension, diabetes, or bleeding problems should start on a much lower dose of vitamin E (100 IU per day) and increase their dosage gradually; if you have any of these conditions, ask your physician about the advisability of these supplements. Otherwise, vitamin E tends to be extremely safe and is commonly used.

Melatonin and 5-Hydroxy Tryptophan. Melatonin is a substance normally produced by our pineal gland that helps to regulate sleep and causes drowsiness. It is produced within the body from the essential amino acid tryptophan, which is then converted into 5-hydroxy tryptophan, serotonin and finally, melatonin. Women with menopause-related insomnia may get some relief by using either **melatonin, 1.5 to 3.0 mg, or 5-hydroxy tryptophan, 50 to 100 mg, taken before bedtime.**

Magnesium. The body requires adequate levels of magnesium in order to maintain energy and vitality. In menopausal women, magnesium is required in order to produce ATP (adenosine triphosphate), the end product of the conversion of food to usable energy by the body's cells. ATP is the universal energy currency the body uses to run hundreds of thousands of chemical reactions. The digestive system can extract this energy from food efficiently only in the presence of magnesium, oxygen and other nutrients. When magnesium is deficient, ATP production falls and the body forms lactic acid instead. Researchers have linked excessive accumulation of lactic acid with anxiety and irritability symptoms.

Magnesium also facilitates conversion of the essential fatty acid linoleic acid to gamma-linolenic acid and its conversion to the beneficial relaxant prostaglandin hormones. These hormones help reduce anxiety and mood-swing symptoms in susceptible women.

Many menopausal women feel depressed and tired due to the chemical and hormonal changes occurring at this time. Medical research studies on the treatment of fatigue use a special form of magnesium called magnesium aspartate, formed by combining magnesium with aspartic acid. Aspartic acid also plays an important role in the production of energy in the body and helps transport magnesium and potassium into the cells. In a number of clinical studies, magnesium aspartate, along with potassium aspartate, has been shown to reduce fatigue after five to six weeks of constant use. Many of those in the study began to feel better after just ten days. This beneficial effect was seen in 90 percent of those tested, a very high success rate.

Magnesium supplements can also benefit women who have menopause-related insomnia. When taken before bedtime, magnesium helps calm the mood and induce restful sleep. Good food sources of magnesium include green leafy vegetables, beans, peas, raw nuts and seeds, tofu, avocados, raisins, dried figs, millet and other grains. **Menopausal women need 400 to 750 mg per day of magnesium, either from food sources or nutritional supplements, for their daily allowance.**

Potassium. Like magnesium, potassium has a powerful enhancing effect on energy and vitality. Potassium deficiency has been associated with fatigue and muscular weakness. One study showed that older people deficient in potassium had weak grip strength. In a number of studies on chronic fatigue, potassium aspartate combined with magnesium aspartate significantly restored energy levels; this combination may be quite useful in menopausal women suffering from excessive fatigue and depression when mineral deficiencies coexist with the lack of hormones.

Potassium can be lost through chronic diarrhea or the overuse of diuretics. In addition, the excessive use of coffee and alcohol (both of which can magnify anxiety and emotional stress symptoms) increase the loss of potassium through the urinary tract.

For women suffering from potassium loss, the use of a potassium supplement may be helpful. The most common dose available is a 99 mg tablet or capsule. I generally recommend one to two per day during times of extreme stress and fatigue. Potassium, however, should be used cautiously. Women with kidney or cardiovascular disease should avoid potassium because high levels can cause an irregular heartbeat. Also, potassium can irritate the intestinal tract, so it should be taken with meals. If you have any questions about the proper use of this mineral, ask your health care provider. Potassium occurs in abundance in fruits, vegetables, beans and peas, seeds and nuts, starches and whole grains.

Calcium. Calcium is the most abundant mineral in the body. This important mineral helps combat stress, nervous tension and anxiety. An upset emotional state can dramatically increase tension and fatigue in susceptible women. A calcium deficiency increases not only emotional irritability but also muscular irritability and cramps. Calcium taken at night along with magnesium will reduce muscular cramps, calm the mood and induce a restful sleep in menopausal women. Women with menopause-related anxiety, mood swings and fatigue may find calcium supplements useful.

Many women consume less than the recommended daily allowance for calcium in their diet (800 mg for women during active reproductive years, 1200 to 1500 mg after menopause). In fact, many women only take in half the recommended amount through diet. In addition, anxiety and stress can inhibit calcium absorption, as will a high-fat diet, lack of exercise and other risk factors. As a result, a calcium supplement may be useful. Good food sources of calcium include green leafy vegetables, salmon (with bones), nuts, seeds, tofu and blackstrap molasses.

Zinc. Zinc is an essential trace mineral necessary for the absorption and assimilation of vitamins, especially the anxiety- and stress-combating B vitamins. It is a constituent of many enzymes involved in metabolism and digestion. Zinc helps reduce anxiety and upset in menopausal women when there is a coexisting blood sugar imbalance. This is due to zinc's role in normal carbohydrate digestion. Because diabetes becomes increasingly prevalent after menopause, support of carbohydrate metabolism is extremely important in midlife women. Zinc is a component of insulin, the protein that helps move glucose out of blood circulation and into the cells. Once inside the cells, glucose provides them with their main source of energy. **Menopausal women may want to use between 15 and 25 mg of zinc per day in a supplemental form.** Good food sources of zinc include soy meal, whole wheat, chicken, rice bran, black-eyed peas, buckwheat, cabbage, pumpkin seeds and peanut butter.

Chromium and Manganese. These two minerals are also important in carbohydrate production metabolism. Chromium helps keep the blood sugar level balanced by enhancing insulin function so that glucose is properly utilized by the body. This avoids the extremes of too little glucose in the blood (hypoglycemia) or too much glucose (diabetes mellitus). Improving the uptake of glucose into the cells allows these cells to use the glucose to produce energy. Manganese aids glucose metabolism by acting as a cofactor in the process of converting glucose (food) to energy.

Good sources of chromium include brewer's yeast (difficult for many women to digest), whole wheat, rye, oysters, potatoes, apples, bananas, spinach, molasses and chicken. Dietary sources of manganese are whole grains, nuts, beans, peas and green leafy vegetables. Many menopausal women (as well as men and women of all ages) lack adequate dietary sources of these nutrients. It is probably a good idea to use a high-potency multivitamin and mineral supplement in order to obtain sufficient amounts of these minerals on a daily basis.

The optimal dosage for Chromium is 150mcg per day and for manganese 4-5 mg per day.

Osteoporosis

Isoflavones. Isoflavones derived from soy should be an important part of the diet of every woman who is at risk for osteoporosis. Soy isoflavones provide many of the same benefits found with conventional hormone therapy but without the side effects and risk factors. Soy isoflavones inhibit the breakdown of bone tissue and improve the bones mineral content, thereby assuring stronger, denser bones. They also promote better calcium circulation by increasing calcium absorption from the intestinal tract, while decreasing calcium loss in the urine. Asian women, whose diets tend to be much richer in soy isoflavones than those of Western women, have a significantly lower risk of fractures due to osteoporosis.

Ipriflavone. This is another isoflavone that has proven useful in the prevention of osteoporosis. While not estrogenic, it has been found to reduce bone loss and maintain bone density in both human and animal studies. **Dosage is 600 mg per day.**

Calcium. Dozens of studies reinforce the importance of calcium for the prevention of osteoporosis. A study reported in the *New England Journal of Medicine* found that women and men aged 65 and older who used calcium and vitamin D supplementation had a lower incidence of bone fracture, as well as reduced loss of bone mass in the hip and spine. This was confirmed at one-year and three-year intervals. Calcium is the most abundant mineral in the body, and 99 percent of it is deposited in the bones and teeth. (The other one percent is involved in blood clotting, nerve and muscle stimulation, and other important functions.)

As a result, calcium is the most important structural mineral in bone. However, calcium absorption becomes much less efficient by the time women reach their postmenopausal years due to aging of the digestive tract. Calcium needs an acid environment in the stomach for proper digestion and, unfortunately, as many as 40 percent of postmenopausal women lack sufficient stomach acid for proper calcium absorption.

The average American woman takes in 400 to 500 mg per day. This is far less than the recommended daily allowance (RDA) of 800 mg per day for women during their active reproductive years and the 1200 to 1500 mg per day needed by postmenopausal women. Both the National Institutes of Health and the National Osteoporosis Foundation recommend that postmenopausal women take 1500 mg daily to compensate for calcium loss. To compound this problem, calcium absorption is inefficient and only 20 to 30 percent of the calcium ingested is utilized by the body.

As a result, adequate calcium supplementation as well as the specific type of calcium used is of major importance for most women. The main type of calcium supplements has been calcium carbonate. This is an alkaline form of calcium and is very good for bone support. Another form is calcium citrate, an acidified form of calcium, is well-absorbed and a good source of the nutrient for women wishing to prevent bone loss.

Phosphorus. Phosphorus is the second most abundant mineral in the body, found in bones and soft tissues. A major structural mineral of bone, it is present in the bones in a specific ratio of 2.5 parts calcium to 1 part phosphorus. This balance is important for both minerals to be used efficiently by the body. Because the American diet contains abundant phosphorus in foods such as meat, eggs, grains, seeds, nuts and soft drinks, phosphorus deficiency is relatively rare. In addition, phosphorus is easily absorbed from the digestive tract with an approximately 70 percent absorption rate. **There is generally no deficiency of phosphorous because it is readily available in our food supply.**

Magnesium. While not as prevalent as either calcium or phosphorus in bone, magnesium is equally important for healthy bones. Mild magnesium deficiency may be a risk factor in the development of osteoporosis. Magnesium is needed for bone growth as well as proper calcium absorption and assimilation. If the body does not have enough magnesium available, calcium can accumulate in the muscles, heart and kidneys (thereby increasing the risk of kidney stones). Calcium and magnesium should be taken in a ratio of 2 to 1 or 10 to 4. Other minerals, such as zinc, copper, manganese and silicon, are also needed in trace amounts for healthy bone growth and regulation of bone metabolism. Because boron is an important trace mineral that has been found to decrease the risk of osteoporosis, mineral supplements developed for this purpose will contain 3 mg of boron per day in their formula.

Vitamins D and K. Vitamin D is a fat soluble vitamin that can either be ingested in the diet or formed on the skin through exposure to sunlight. Sunlight activates a type of cholesterol found in the skin, converting it to vitamin D.

Vitamin D helps prevent osteoporosis by aiding in the absorption of calcium from the intestinal tract. It is needed for the synthesis of enzymes found in mucous membranes that are used in the active transport of calcium.

Vitamin D also helps break down and assimilate phosphorus. A deficiency of vitamin D causes inadequate absorption of calcium from the intestinal tract as well as retention of phosphorus by the kidneys. This causes an imbalance in the calcium-phosphorus ratio, leading to faulty mineralization of the bones. Vitamin D is usually included in multivitamin products and is also found in fish liver oil supplements (along with vitamin A) and fortified milk. Menopausal women should have at least 1000-2000 IU per day of vitamin D.

Vitamin K is a fat soluble vitamin stored in your body in the fatty tissues and liver. It is found abundantly in leafy green vegetables. Vitamin K is necessary to help calcium build bone. Women with higher levels of vitamin K have higher bone density and improved bone health. Dosage is 100-200 mcg of vitamin K.

Cardiovascular Disease

Isoflavones. An analysis of thirty-eight studies conducted on the use of soy protein (a rich source of isoflavones) in the reduction of elevated cholesterol levels (a major risk factor for heart attacks and strokes) found that the daily consumption of 50 grams of soy protein was quite effective. Total cholesterol levels were reduced by nearly 10 percent. Equally impressive were reductions in LDL cholesterol and triglycerides. (Fifty grams of soy protein is slightly less than two ounces.)

Beta-Carotene. Oxygen-related damage to LDL cholesterol has been linked to the development of cardiovascular disease. Laboratory and clinical studies suggest that beta carotene can prevent this oxygen-related damage, a process that can initiate atherogenesis (the destruction of the blood vessel wall and the formation of plaque) and eventually cause heart attacks and strokes. Beta-carotene can thereby help protect the blood vessels from the disease process. *The U.S. Physicians' Health Study* found in a group of 333 participants with chest pain, but no prior history of heart attack, that beta carotene appeared to have a protective effect. Fifty percent fewer major cardiovascular events occurred, including heart attacks, strokes and cardiac related deaths. **I recommend 5,000 to 20,000 IU of beta-carotene per day.**

Vitamin C. Like beta-carotene, vitamin C is a water-soluble vitamin that appears to be helpful in preventing LDL cholesterol oxidation, a process that can initiate atherogenesis. In *The Nurses Health Study*, in which over 87,000 women between the ages of 34 and 54 were studied, the association between dietary intake of vitamin C and the risk of developing coronary artery disease was evaluated. The risk of developing heart disease was more than 42 percent lower for women who used high doses of vitamin C than for women with a low vitamin C intake. Another study in Boston found that both males and females using vitamin C supplementation had lower levels of blood pressure, lower LDL cholesterol and higher HDL cholesterol (the type of cholesterol that confers protection against coronary artery disease) than participants with a lower vitamin C intake. Vitamin C is also necessary for the regeneration of vitamin E in the body, another important antioxidant nutrient. These results make a good case for vitamin C cardiovascular protective effects.

A dose between 1000 and 5000 mg of mineral buffered vitamin C per day taken in divided doses can be quite useful for its protective effects on the body. Good food sources of vitamin C include many fruits and vegetables.

Vitamin E. Vitamin E completes the triumvirate of antioxidant vitamins that appear to confer protection against cardiovascular disease. Two major studies of health care professionals, done at Brigham and Women's Hospital and the Harvard School of Public Health in Boston, confirm other studies by the World Health Organization that low levels of vitamin E are a more important predictor of ischemic heart disease than high cholesterol levels. This protective effect is seen with intake of more than 100 IUs per day. Vitamin E is the main fat-soluble antioxidant nutrient in the body. It lodges within the membranes inside and surrounding the cells, protecting the body against attack by singlet (unstable) oxygen and other free radicals that cause cell destruction. As mentioned earlier, singlet oxygen or other free-radical destruction of LDL cholesterol may be one of the early steps leading to atherogenesis and ultimately cardiovascular disease. Vitamin E, along with beta-carotene and vitamin C, provides protection for both the water compartment and the fat compartment of our cells. This is necessary for the most complete protection against oxidative damage. Vitamin E also has a beneficial anticlotting effect on the blood. While a high saturated fat diet tends to cause blood cells to clump together, vitamin E helps prevent this by causing the cells to disperse. This helps prevent blood clots from forming. **I recommend 800 to 1600 IU of natural vitamin E per day.**

Essential Fatty Acids. The supplemental use of Omega-3 fatty acids derived from fish, such as salmon, trout and halibut as well as plants, such as flaxseeds, pumpkin seeds and soy beans, have certain protective effects against cardiovascular disease. In a number of medical studies, Omega-3 fatty acids have been shown to inhibit platelet cell aggregation (important in preventing clot formation) as well as relaxing and dilating the blood vessels. In addition, Omega-3 fatty acids lower the level of triglycerides; this is beneficial because elevated levels of triglycerides are a risk factor for coronary artery disease.

While they can help lower the level of triglycerides, the benefits for reducing LDL cholesterol are not as clear cut. Also, because fish oil consumption can create a moderate reduction in blood pressure in people with hypertension. **I recommend 2000 to 3000 mg of fish oil capsules containing EPA (eicosapentaenoic acid) and DHA (docosahexaenoic acid) per day.**

Breast Cancer

Isoflavones. An analysis of thirty studies published explored the relationship between soy-based diets and cancer. The soy-based diets were found to dramatically reduce the incidence of breast, prostate and uterine cancers. Asian women who consumed a soy-based diet were four to six times less likely to have breast cancer compared to women in the United States who consumed the standard American diet, which contains virtually no isoflavones. **I recommend 50 to 100 mg of isoflavones per day.**

Vitamin A. Beta-carotene has been cited in a number of studies as being an important nutrient in breast cancer prevention. *The Nurses Health Study* sponsored by Harvard University, which looked at the health and lifestyle habits of over 87,000 women, found that beta carotene, indeed, had a protective effect. Another study published by the State University of New York, compared 310 women having breast cancer to 316 women without the disease. The study found that the cancer-free group consumed many more beta carotene-containing fruits and vegetables than the women with breast cancer. Both beta-carotene in supplemental form, as well as abundant fresh fruits and vegetables, should be included in your diet if you are concerned about breast cancer prevention. **I recommend 5000 to 20,000 IU of beta-carotene per day taken as a supplement.**

Vitamin C. In a review of 46 studies of the protective effect of vitamin C on cancer, the results of 33 studies showed that vitamin C helped safeguard against the development of many cancers; this included nonhormone-dependent breast cancer. Vitamin C did not appear to confer any protection against hormone-dependent (including estrogen-dependent) breast cancers.

Because fruits and vegetables are rich sources of both beta carotene and vitamin C, they are ideal sources of these nutrients. Women who wish to lower their cancer risk for all types of cancer (including certain breast cancers) may also want to use supplemental vitamin C. **I recommend 1000 to 3000 mg of buffered vitamin C taken in divided doses per day.**

Vitamin and Mineral Supplements for Women in Midlife

Good dietary habits are crucial for control of your menopause symptoms. But for many women, the use of nutritional supplements is important in order to achieve high levels of the essential nutrients needed to relieve their symptoms. On the following pages is a sample of the vitamins and minerals as well as their dosages that can be used as a foundation for your program. You can also add the other nutrients like flaxseed oil and fish oil that I have discussed in this chapter to fill out your program.

You may find it easier to implement your program if you start with one of the better quality multi-nutrient products for women that are available in health food stores and through the Internet and then add the remaining essential nutrients.

Remember that all women differ somewhat in their nutritional needs. If you do take the recommended vitamin or herbal supplements, I usually advise that you start with one-fourth to one-half the dose recommended in this book and work your way up slowly to the higher dosage, if needed. You may find that you do best with slightly more or less of certain ingredients.

I recommend that patients take their supplements with meals or at least a snack. Very rarely, a woman will have a digestive reaction to supplements, such as nausea or indigestion. If this happens, stop all supplements; then resume using them, adding one at a time, until you find the offending nutrient. Eliminate from your program any nutrient to which you have a reaction. If you have any specific questions, ask a health-care professional who is knowledgeable about nutrition.

Optimal Nutritional Supplementation for Menopause

Vitamins and Minerals	Maximum Daily Dosage
Vitamin A	5000 I.U.
Beta carotene (provitamin A)	10,000 – 25,000 I.U.
Vitamin B complex	
B1 (thiamine)	25 - 100 mg
B2 (riboflavin)	25 - 100 mg
B3 (niacinamide)	25 - 100 mg
B5 (pantothenic acid)	25 - 100 mg
B6 (pyridoxine)	50 – 100 mg
B12 (cyanocobalamin)	250– 750 mcg
Folic acid	400 – 800 mcg
Biotin	200 - 500 mcg
Choline	25 - 100 mg
Inositol	25 - 100 mg
PABA	50 - 400 mg
Vitamin C (as mineral ascorbates)	1000-2000 mg
Vitamin D	1000 I.U.
Bioflavonoids	800-2000 mg
Rutin	200 mg
Vitamin E (d-alpha tocopherol acetate)	800-1600 I.U.
Calcium	1000 - 1200 mg
Magnesium	500 - 600 mg
Potassium	100 mg
Iron	18 mg
Zinc	15 mg
Iodine	150 mcg
Manganese	5 mg
Copper	2 mg
Selenium	200 mcg
Chromium	100 – 200 mcg
Boron	3 mg

Food Sources of Vitamin A

Vegetables
Carrots
Carrot juice
Collard greens
Dandelion greens
Green onions
Kale
Parsley
Spinach
Sweet potatoes
Turnip greens
Winter squash

Fruits
Apricots
Avocado
Cantaloupe
Mangoes
Papaya
Peaches
Persimmons

Meat, poultry, seafood
Crab
Halibut
Liver—all types
Mackerel
Salmon

Food Sources of Vitamin B Complex (including folic acid)

Vegetables
Alfalfa
Artichoke
Asparagus
Beets
Broccoli
Brussels sprouts
Cabbage
Cauliflower
Green beans
Kale
Leeks
Onions
Peas
Romaine lettuce

Legumes
Garbanzo beans
Lentils
Lima beans
Pinto beans
Soybeans

Meat, poultry, seafood
Egg yolks*
Liver*

*Eggs and meat should be from organic, free-range stock fed on pesticide-free food.

Grains
Barley
Bran
Brown rice
Corn Millet
Rice bran
Wheat
Wheat germ

Sweeteners
Blackstrap molasses

Food Sources of Vitamin B6

Grains
Brown rice
Buckwheat flour
Rice bran
Rye flour
Wheat germ
Whole wheat flour

Vegetables
Asparagus
Beet greens
Broccoli
Brussels sprouts
Cauliflower
Green peas
Leeks
Sweet potatoes

Meat, poultry, seafood
Chicken
Salmon
Shrimp
Tuna

Nuts and seeds
Sunflower seeds

Food Sources of Vitamin C

Fruits
Blackberries
Black currants
Cantaloupe
Elderberries
Grapefruit
Grapefruit juice
Guavas
Kiwi fruit
Mangoes
Oranges
Orange juice
Pineapple
Raspberries
Strawberries
Tangerines
Tomatoes

Vegetables and legumes
Asparagus
Black-eyed peas
Broccoli
Brussels sprouts
Cabbage
Cauliflower
Collards
Green onions
Green peas
Kale
Kohlrabi
Parsley
Potatoes
Rutabagas
Sweet pepper
Sweet potatoes
Turnips

Meat, poultry, seafood
Liver—all types
Pheasant
Quail
Salmon

Food Sources of Vitamin E

Vegetables
Asparagus
Cucumber
Green peas
Kale

Meats, poultry, seafood
Haddock
Herring
Mackerel
Lamb
Liver—all types

Grains
Brown rice
Millet

Nuts and seeds
Almonds
Brazil nuts
Hazelnuts
Peanuts

Oils
Corn
Peanut
Safflower
Sesame
Soybean
Wheat germ

Fruits
Mangoes

Food Sources of Essential Fatty Acids

Flaxseeds
Pumpkin seeds
Soybeans
Walnuts
Safflower oil

Sunflower oil
Sesame seeds

Food Sources of Iron

Grains
Bran cereal (All-Bran)
Bran muffin
Millet, dry
Oat flakes
Pasta, whole wheat
Pumpernickel bread
Wheat germ

Vegetables
Beets
Beet greens
Broccoli
Brussels sprouts
Corn
Dandelion greens
Green beans
Kale
Leeks
Spinach
Sweet potatoes
Swiss chard

Meat, poultry, seafood
Beef liver
Calf's liver
Chicken liver
Clams
Oysters
Sardines
Scallops
Trout

Legumes
Black beans
Black-eyed peas
Garbanzo beans
Kidney beans
Lentils
Lima beans
Pinto beans
Soybeans
Split peas
Tofu

Fruits
Apple juice
Avocado
Blackberries
Dates, dried
Figs
Prunes, dried
Prune juice
Raisins

Nuts and seeds
Almonds
Pecans
Pistachios
Sesame butter
Sesame seeds
Sunflower seeds

Food Sources of Calcium

Vegetables and legumes
Artichoke
Black beans
Black-eyed peas
Beet greens
Broccoli
Brussels sprouts
Cabbage
Collards
Eggplant
Garbanzo beans
Green beans
Green onions
Kale
Kidney beans
Leeks
Lentils
Parsley
Parsnips
Pinto beans
Rutabagas
Soybeans
Spinach
Turnips
Watercress

Meat, poultry, seafood
Abalone
Beef
Bluefish
Carp
Crab
Haddock
Herring
Lamb
Lobster
Oysters
Perch
Salmon
Shrimp
Venison

Fruits
Blackberries
Black currants
Boysenberries
Oranges
Pineapple juice
Prunes
Raisins
Rhubarb
Tangerine juice

Grains
Bran
Brown rice
Bulgar wheat
Millet

Food Sources of Magnesium

Vegetables and legumes
Artichoke
Black-eyed peas
Carrot juice
Corn
Green peas
Leeks
Lima beans
Okra
Parsnips
Potatoes
Soybean sprouts
Spinach
Squash
Yams
Snapper
Turkey
Papaya

Meat, poultry, seafood
Beef
Carp
Chicken
Clams
Cod
Crab
Duck
Haddock
Herring
Lamb
Mackerel
Oysters
Salmon
Shrimp
Raisins
Prunes

Nuts and seeds
Almonds
Brazil nuts
Hazelnuts
Peanuts
Pistachios
Pumpkin seeds
Sesame seeds
Walnuts

Fruits
Avocado
Banana
Grapefruit juice
Pineapple juice

Grains
Millet
Brown rice
Wild rice

Food Sources of Potassium

Vegetables and legumes
Artichoke
Asparagus
Black-eyed peas
Beets
Brussels sprouts
Carrot juice
Cauliflower
Corn
Garbanzo beans
Green beans
Kidney beans
Leeks
Lentils
Lima beans
Navy beans
Okra
Parsnips
Peas
Pinto beans
Potatoes
Pumpkin
Soybean sprouts
Spinach
Squash
Yams

Meat, poultry, seafood
Bass
Beef
Carp
Catfish
Chicken
Cod
Duck
Eel
Flatfish
Haddock
Halibut
Herring
Lamb
Lobster
Mackerel
Oysters
Perch
Pike
Salmon
Scallops
Shrimp
Snapper
Trout
Turkey
Raisins

Nuts and seeds
Almonds
Brazil nuts
Chestnuts
Hazelnuts
Macadamia nuts
Peanuts
Pistachios
Pumpkin seeds
Sesame seeds
Sunflower seeds
Walnuts

Fruits
Apricots
Avocado
Banana
Cantaloupe
Currants
Figs
Grapefruit juice
Orange juice
Papaya
Pineapple juice
Prunes

Grains
Brown rice
Millet
Wild rice

Food Sources of Zinc

Grains

Barley
Brown rice
Buckwheat
Corn
Cornmeal
Millet
Oatmeal
Rice bran
Rye bread
Wheat bran
Wheat germ
Wheat berries
Whole wheat bread
Whole wheat flour

Vegetables and Legumes

Black-eyed peas
Cabbage
Carrots
Garbanzo beans
Green peas
Lentils
Lettuce
Lima beans
Onions
Soy flour
Soy meal
Soy protein

Fruits

Apples
Peaches

Meat, Poultry, Seafood

Chicken
Oysters

17

Herbs That Relieve Specific Symptoms of Menopause

Herbs have a long and distinguished history for the treatment of female complaints. Plant-based remedies were our first real medicines; the history of their use spans thousands of years. An understanding of their healing properties was based on observation as well as trial and error. Valuable research on medicinal benefits of plants continues today, using modern scientific techniques of testing and analysis.

Herbs can help balance and expand the diet while optimizing nutritional intake. If you are interested in using herbs, try them as a part of your menopause relief nutritional program.

Herbs For Menopause

This section provides information on herbs that can help relieve menopause related symptoms. Many women have found helpful and effective herbal remedies for the relief of common menopausal symptoms. These remedies, along with a healthy diet, are a form of extended nutrition.

Heavy or Irregular Menstrual Bleeding

Heavy or irregular menstrual bleeding is a common problem experienced by women progressing into menopause. Luckily, many bioflavonoid containing plants can help smooth out menstrual irregularities and reduce the quantity of blood lost during this time of hormonal instability. They do this in two ways. Plants containing bioflavonoids strengthen the capillaries and help prevent them from rupturing, thereby reducing blood loss. In addition, bioflavonoids are weakly estrogenic, as well as anti-estrogenic. Because they compete with estrogen precursors in the body for binding sites on enzymes, they help reduce your own levels of estrogen, which can be quite high during the menopause transition period. This reduces estrogen stimulation to the uterine lining, decreasing the amount of blood flow that can occur with menstruation. Citrus bioflavonoids are the most commonly available type of bioflavonoid found in health food stores. **I usually recommend 1000 to 2000 mg per day with an equal amount of mineral buffered vitamin C.**

Good food sources of bioflavonoids include citrus fruits, bilberries, cherries, and grape skins. Bioflavonoids have also been found in red clover and in some clover strains in Australia. Many of these plants are available as herbal tinctures (liquid) or in capsules and can be taken in supplemental form.

Two herbs that women have traditionally used to stop excessive menstrual flow and postpartum hemorrhage are golden seal and shepherd's purse. Golden seal contains a chemical called berberine that calms uterine muscular tension. (It has also been used to calm and soothe the digestive tract.) Shepherd's purse helps promote blood clotting and has been used to help stop menstrual bleeding. However, if your bleeding is excessive or irregular, consult your physician. This should be evaluated carefully by your physician and, if necessary, medical therapy should be instituted. Excessive and irregular bleeding can be dangerous and should never be allowed to continue without medical help. Women with a normal menstrual flow that is somewhat heavier may find the mild properties of herbs helpful for symptom relief.

Other herbs help prevent iron-deficiency anemia that can result from heavy menstrual flow during the early menopause period. These herbs provide good sources of nonheme iron. Outstanding examples are yellow dock and pau d'arco. Yellow dock is also used to help promote liver health, which is important in the regulation of estrogen levels because the liver breaks down estrogen and prepares it for excretion from the body. When estrogen levels are too high, heavy menstrual bleeding can occur. Turmeric, or curcuma, is also used to promote liver health in traditional medicine. Recent research suggests that it has antibacterial and anti-inflammatory properties. Turmeric is an herb often used for flavoring in traditional Indian dishes. Silymarin, or milk thistle, contains strong antioxidants that protect the liver from damage.

Hot Flashes, Night Sweats, Vaginal and Bladder Atrophy

Phytoestrogen plants abound in nature. These plants contain natural sources of estrogen, similar to that manufactured by our own body. Many of these plants can be used as an estrogen substitute by women who cannot or do not want to use estrogen in pharmacological dosages. For women who have pre-existing health problems, such as migraine headaches or hypertension, or who are sensitive to the dosages used in standard replacement therapy, phytoestrogen herbs provide a helpful alternative.

Compared with drug potencies, plant sources of estrogen are very weak. Other estrogen-containing plants such as fennel, anise and black cohosh, have been assayed as 1/400 the potency of estradiol, the main form of estrogen made by the ovaries. Because of their low potencies, estrogen-containing herbs tend to have a low potential for causing side effects, yet are quite effective in suppressing such common menopause symptoms as hot flashes and night sweats. They can even help build up the vaginal lining.

The most widely studied phytoestrogen is black cohosh. An article in the *American Journal of Natural Medicine* reviewed the studies to date on black cohosh. These studies found that it produced better results than conventional therapies such as Premarin, Valium and other hormonal and mood-altering drugs in relieving menopausal hot flashes, vaginal atrophy and mood swings, and without increasing the risk of uterine or breast cancer.

Plants may also form the basis for the production of medical hormones. Soy beans and wild yams contain a preformed steroidal nucleus. Estrogen and progesterone can be synthesized from these plants in relatively few steps; this has allowed sex hormones to become available commercially at reasonable cost. For many years it was believed that wild yam (which comes from the barbasco root, a giant, wild yam found in Mexico), converted to DHEA in the body. But current research has shown that this is not the case.

Women who suffer from vaginal and bladder atrophy due to estrogen deficiency run the additional risk of increased incidence of infections in these tissues after menopause. Many herbs can soothe, relieve irritation, and reduce infection in the urinary tract; these include golden seal, uva ursi, blackberry root, and wintergreen. Golden seal contains berberine, an alkaloid with antibiotic activity that may help suppress urinary tract infections.

Menopause Related Insomnia

Kava root has been used for centuries in the Pacific Islands to encourage a greater sense of well-being and relaxation at ceremonial events. Kava is currently being used in the West for the treatment of insomnia. **I recommend 140 to 210 mg one hour before bedtime.**

Passionflower has been found to elevate levels of the neurotransmitter serotonin. Serotonin is synthesized from tryptophan, an essential amino acid that has been shown in numerous medical studies to initiate restful sleep. Valerian root has been used extensively in traditional herbal medicine as a sleep inducer, and is widely used both in Europe and the United States as a gentle herbal remedy to help combat insomnia. Unfortunately, valerian has an unpleasant taste, which is more palatable when used in capsule form.

Many women with moderate to severe symptoms of hormonal deficiency wake up two to three times a night. If you suffer from menopause-related insomnia, you may need to make a fairly strong sedative tea such as hops or chamomile, using two or three tea bags instead of one. Start with a weaker tea and increase the potency slowly until you find the level that works best for you.

Many menopausal women also suffer from the unpleasant physical symptoms of tight, tense muscles in vulnerable areas of their bodies (neck, shoulders, and jaw, as well as the upper and lower back, are common areas to store tension). Many of these relaxant herbs help relieve the muscle tension and spasm that often accompanies stress. Valerian root, peppermint, and chamomile also relieve stress-related indigestion and intestinal gas.

Menopause Anxiety, Irritability and Insomnia

Specific herbs can provide helpful relief for the emotional symptoms of menopause. Plants such as kava, valerian root, passionflower, hops, chamomile and skullcap have a significant calming and restful effect on the central nervous system. Clinical studies confirm that kava is particularly helpful in reducing symptoms of anxiety and stress. They all promote emotional calm and well-being. With their mild sedative effect, they also promote restful sleep, a difficult state to induce in a woman suffering from menopause-related insomnia.

Menopause-related Fatigue and Depression

Menopausal women commonly suffer from depression and fatigue. Sometimes these symptoms co-exist with anxiety and irritability. Menopausal women with mood swings that vacillate between highs and lows often feel that they are on an emotional roller coaster.

Kava, in particular, can help when feelings of anxiety and depression coexist. St. Johns wort is another herb that has been studied for its mood-altering effects. Extract of St. Johns wort, standardized to 0.3 hypericin (the active ingredient) has been found to have significant antidepressant benefits without the side effects frequently seen with medication. Herbs such as oat straw, ginger, ginkgo biloba, dandelion root and Siberian ginseng (eleutherococcus) also have a stimulatory effect, improving energy and vitality. Women who use these herbs may note an increased ability to handle stress, as well as improved physical and mental capabilities.

Siberian ginseng and ginger have been used in traditional Asian medicines to increase longevity and decrease fatigue and weakness. These herbs boost immunity and strengthen the cardiovascular system. The bioflavonoids contained in ginkgo are extremely powerful antioxidants and help to combat fatigue by improving circulation to the brain. They may also improve the function of the adrenal and thyroid glands. Oat straw has also been used to relieve fatigue and weakness.

In modern China, Japan and other countries, there is a great deal of interest in the pharmacological effects of these traditional herbs. Scientific studies are corroborating the medicinal effects of these plants.

Osteoporosis, Heart Disease and Breast Disease

Herbs can provide a valuable source of minerals along with other foods in the diet. Certain plants, such as kelp and other sea vegetables, as well as dandelion root, horsetail, and oat straw are good sources of calcium, magnesium, and trace minerals needed for strong and healthy bones. Kelp and the other sea vegetables can be used as condiments to flavor food such as soups, casseroles, and salads. The other herbs may be taken in capsule form as a supplement.

Garlic and ginger are two delicious herbs that are used commonly as flavoring agents. They are also beneficial in reducing the risk of heart disease. These two plants should be used frequently as part of your preventative program if you have a strong family history of heart disease with early mortality (parents or siblings dying in their 50s or 60s of heart disease). They should also be used if you have any risk factors yourself, such as hypertension or elevated cholesterol. Both garlic and ginger have been researched for their ability to prevent aggregation, or clotting, of the blood. This is important for the prevention of strokes and heart attacks. In addition, both herbs help reduce cholesterol levels. Garlic has the additional benefit of reducing blood pressure. However, your physician may recommend avoiding the use of these herbs in supplemental form if you are taking blood-thinning medication like Coumadin. Small amounts in cooking may be ok.

If you find these foods too spicy for your taste buds, they can be used in capsule form or as a liquid tincture. Women using these herbs for cardio-vascular disease prevention may want to eat several raw cloves of garlic a day or take as many as six capsules of the herb as a supplement. I also recommend as many as four capsules of ginger per day, if you do not use it as a food flavoring. These are maximum dosages; you may find that one to two capsules per day suit your needs better.

Many herbs show promise in the prevention or treatment of many human cancers, although their specific role in treating breast cancer is not clear. Herbs with possible anticancer activity include garlic, burdock root, alfalfa and a host of others. One herb in particular may hold some promise for breast cancer prevention. This is red clover, an herb traditionally used by several different cultures to treat cancer. Research done at the National Cancer Institute has found anticarcinogenic compounds in red clover, including several bioflavonoids, genistein and daidzein, which are both weakly estrogenic and anti-estrogenic. Women with a pre-existing breast cancer may want to check with their physician to see if red clover can be used safely as a nutritional adjunct to their regular medical program.

Herbal Formulas for Women in Midlife

Herbs are an effective means of balancing the diet and optimizing nutritional intake. Herbal products should be used in small amounts and taken with your meals in either capsule form or in a tea. If you buy a commercial product, do not take more than the recommended dosage of the herbal mix. If you prefer to make a tea, simply empty the capsule into a cup of boiling water and let it steep for a few minutes. Do not drink more than one or two cups of the tea per day.

All foods have the potential for causing distress in some people and herbs are no exception. They should be discontinued immediately if you experience nausea, vomiting or diarrhea after use. These are the most common symptoms of intolerance. The herbs in my formulas are all recommended as being safe for human consumption, but rarely a woman may react adversely to various foods, including herbs. If you notice any symptoms that make you uncomfortable after using the herbs, discontinue them immediately.

18

Stress Reduction for Menopause

Menopause may be a time of mood swings and emotional upset for many women. This can occur both during the transition towards menopause and the early postmenopausal years. Often, these emotional changes are due to the instability in the female hormones, estrogen and progesterone, as they readjust to a new and lower level of equilibrium. Both estrogen and progesterone affect brain chemistry (progesterone has a sedative effect and estrogen acts as a brain stimulant); therefore, their fluctuating levels can wreak havoc on both mood and body. Emotional symptoms of menopause can include anxiety, irritability, emotional fragility, anger, depression, crying easily, and fatigue. Also, when hot flashes occur at night, they are often linked to insomnia. Severity of these symptoms will vary amongst women due to differences in individual biochemistry as well as stressful and aggravating social factors. Some women go through menopause with no mood changes at all, feeling calm and relaxed. Other women have moderate to severe symptoms, which can be incapacitating, interfering with their quality of life.

For many women, the social and cultural factors occurring around the time of menopause can be as significant as hormonal changes in determining their emotional state. Menopause can be a time of loss, with parents dying or ill, children leaving home, and careers or marriages ending. Often, the old familiar guideposts that have provided stability during the first half of life disappear, leaving a woman feeling lost. On the positive side, it can also be a time of rebirth for the woman and a time of forging or solidifying her own identity. The rebirth process can be difficult and take years to complete. Thus, for many women, the combination of hormonal and biochemical changes plus the social factors can be quite difficult to handle.

Some women require counseling and medication in order to cope with menopause-related emotional symptoms. All women can benefit from self-help techniques such as stress reduction and relaxation exercises. Since the physical, chemical, and social changes are unavoidable, practicing these types of techniques on a regular basis can help bring a sense of peace, calm and stability to your life.

The rest of this chapter is divided into three sections: stress-reduction exercises you can use for general relaxation, for specific premenopause symptoms, and for menopause-related symptoms. Each section contains many different types of exercises so that you can find the ones that work best for you. Try the relaxation techniques that pertain to your symptoms; enjoy the many emotional and physical benefits they bring over time.

Before you begin the exercises, separate yourself physically and mentally from your normal day-to-day environment. At home, find a quiet place where you can be alone. At work, close the door to your office while you take a relaxation break. Many women find that quiet background music promotes a sense of peace as they exercise. Classical music or environmental sounds such as ocean waves or the sound of rain can be very relaxing. In some exercises you sit upright in a comfortable position; in others, the exercises are performed while lying on your back. In either case, your arms and legs should be uncrossed. It is important that your clothes be loose and comfortable. Before you begin each exercise, close your eyes and take a few deep breaths in and out. This will help quiet your mind and remove your thoughts from the tasks of the day.

General Relaxation Exercises

I recommend beginning each stress-reduction session with some general relaxation exercises. These exercises will help you make the transition from your normal busy schedule and day-to-day activities. As you begin to unwind, you will become more receptive to the specific stress-reduction exercises for premenopause and menopause symptoms. The general relaxation exercises also promote good health and well-being for the entire body. You may want to practice them when you feel like taking a quick break during the busy times of the day. The exercises will give you a pick-me-up when your energy starts to wane and your mental edge begins to feel dull. They should rapidly begin to energize and revitalize you.

Exercise 1: Deep Abdominal Breathing

Abdominal breathing is a very important technique for inducing a state of peace and relaxation as well as improving energy and vitality. These can be very valuable goals for women when their physical and emotional well-being is impaired by the chemical and physiological instability of midlife. Deep, slow breathing brings adequate oxygen, the fuel for metabolic activity, to all the tissues of your body. In contrast, the rapid, shallow breathing that occurs during times of stress decreases the oxygen supply, keeping you tired and energy-depleted. Deep breathing helps release tension and anxiety and relaxes the entire body. It also helps balance many other important physiological processes such as pulse rate and hormonal output, thereby improving health.

- Lie flat on your back with your knees pulled up, keeping your feet slightly apart. Try to breathe in and out through your nose.

- Inhale deeply. As you breathe in, allow your stomach to relax so the air flows into your abdomen. Your stomach should balloon out as you breathe in. Visualize your lungs filling with air so your chest swells out.

- Imagine that the air you breathe is filling your body with energy.

- Exhale deeply. As you breathe out, let your stomach and chest collapse. Image the air being pushed out, first from your abdomen and then from your lungs.

- Repeat this exercise 10 times.

Exercise 2: Focusing

- Sit upright in a comfortable position.

- Hold a small, sentimental object in the palm of your hand.

- Focus all of your attention on this object as you inhale and exhale deeply for one to two minutes. Don't let any other thoughts enter your mind.

- At the end of this time, notice your breathing. You should find that it has slowed down and is calm. You will probably feel a sense of peacefulness and a decrease in any stress or tension that you started with when beginning this exercise.

The next three exercises help you identify your areas of muscle tension and then teach you how to release this tension. This is an important sequence for women in transition, menopause, or post menopause who suffer from heavy menstrual flow, blood clots, recurrent menstrual cramps, low back pain, or vaginal and bladder atrophy. Many of these symptoms increase when women localize tension and stress to their pelvic area. Chronically tight and tense muscles in the low back and pelvic region can intensify menopause symptoms. Tense muscles tend to have decreased blood circulation and oxygenation, and may accumulate an excess of waste products, such as carbon dioxide and lactic acid.

Interestingly, many women (and men) tend to tighten and contract certain muscle groups as a habitual reaction to strong emotional patterns. For example, if a person has difficulty expressing feelings verbally, the neck muscles may become chronically tight. A person with repressed anger may have chest pain and tight chest muscles. Many women tend to tighten the pelvis and lower abdominal muscles as a stress response to a variety of work, relationship, and sexual stresses. Usually, the tensing of pelvic muscles is an unconscious response that develops over many years and sets up the emotional patterning that triggers pelvic tension-related symptoms. For example, when a woman has uncomfortable feelings about sex or a particular sexual partner, she may tighten these muscles when engaging in, or even thinking about, sex. Tense muscles can affect a woman's moods, making her more "uptight" and irritable.

Movement through stretching or exercise is one effective way of breaking up these habitual patterns of muscle tensing and contracting. When muscles are loose and limber, a woman will feel more relaxed and in a better mood. Tension and stress fades away, replaced by a sense of expansiveness. The following exercise will help you release tension in your tight muscle groups.

Exercise 3: Discovering Muscle Tension

- Lie on your back in a comfortable position. Allow your arms to rest comfortably at your sides, palms down, on the surface next to you.

- Raise your right arm straight up and hold it elevated for 15 seconds.

- Notice if your forearm feels tight and tense or if the muscles are soft and pliable.

- Let your arm drop down and relax. The arm muscles will relax, too.

- As you lie quietly, notice any other parts of your body that feel tense, muscles that feel tight and sore. You may feel a constant dull aching in certain muscles. Tense muscles block blood flow and cut off the supply of nutrients to the tissues. In response to the poor oxygenation, the muscle produces lactic acid, which further increases muscular discomfort.

- Release the tension in any tense or aching muscles.

Exercise 4: Progressive Muscle Relaxation

- Lie on your back in a comfortable position. Allow your arms to rest at your sides, palms down, on the surface next to you.

- Inhale slowly and deeply through your nose and exhale slowly through your mouth.

- Clench your hands into fists and hold them tightly for 15 seconds. Visualize your fists contracting, becoming tighter and tighter. As you do this, relax the rest of your body.

- Let your hands relax. As you relax, visualize a golden light flowing into the entire body, making all your muscles soft and pliable.

- Now, tense and relax the following parts of your body in this order: face, shoulders, back, stomach, pelvis, legs, feet, and toes. Hold each part tensed for 15 seconds and then relax your body for 30 seconds before going on to the next part.

- Finish the exercise by shaking your hands and imagining the remaining tension flowing out of your fingertips.

Exercise 5: Release of Muscle Tension and Anxiety

- Lie in a comfortable position. Allow your arms to rest at your sides, palms down. Inhale and exhale slowly and deeply with your eyes closed.

- Become aware of your feet, ankles, and legs. Notice whether parts of your body have any muscle tension or tightness. If so, how does the tense part of your body feel? Is it in a viselike grip, knotted, cold, and numb? Do you notice any strong feelings, such as hurt, upset, or anger in that part of your body? Breathe into that part of your body until you feel it relax. Release any anxious feelings with your breathing, continuing until they begin to decrease in intensity and fade.

- Next, move your awareness into your hips, pelvis, and lower back. Note any tension or anxious feelings located in that part of your body. Breathe into your hips and pelvis until you feel them relax. Release any negative emotions as you breathe in and out.

- Focus on your abdomen and chest. Notice any anxious feelings located in this area and let them drop away as you breathe in and out. Continue to release any upsetting feelings located in your abdomen or chest.

- Finally, focus on your head, neck, arms, and hands. Note any tension in this area and release it. With your breathing, release any negative feelings blocked in this area until they disappear.

- When you have finished releasing tension throughout the body, continue deep breathing and relaxing for another minute or two. At the end of this exercise, you should feel lighter and more energized.

Stress Reduction Exercises for Premenopause

The premenopause time can be marked by symptoms of easily triggered feelings such as anxiety, irritability, mood swings, and depression. Physical symptoms include menstrual periods becoming irregular and menstrual flow either more excessive or diminished. In addition, fibroid tumors that have a potential for growing into large ovarian cysts are fairly common and PMS symptoms intensify. Clearly, many women experience this as a stressful time.

The next two exercises help create an easier and less traumatic menopause transition by promoting a positive body—mind interaction. Since the mind, in part, affects the body's level of functioning, positive messages and visual pictures about your changing body can promote optimal health and well-being during this time. Positive mental messages can help reduce symptoms and smooth out the stress inherent in this time of change.

Exercise 6: Affirmations for Premenopause

Affirmations are positive statements that describe how you want your body to be. They are very important because they align your mind with your body in a positive way. Affirmations accomplish this through the power of suggestion. Your state of health is determined, in part, by the thousands of mental messages you send yourself each day. You can aggravate your premenopause symptoms such as excessive bleeding and cramps due to fibroid tumors or anovulatory periods (menstrual cycles when you don't produce progesterone), or even PMS symptoms, with negative thoughts. When your body believes it is sick, it behaves accordingly. It is essential that you cultivate a positive belief system and a positive body image as part of your healing program. It is not enough to follow an excellent diet and a vigorous exercise routine when you are in the process of reducing premenopausal symptoms. You must also tell your body that it is a well, fully functional system. I have seen people remain ill by sabotaging their healing program when they send themselves a barrage of negative messages.

- Sit in a comfortable position. Repeat the following affirmations, repeating three times those that are particularly important to you.

- My female system is strong and healthy.

- My hormonal levels are perfectly balanced and regulated.

- My body chemistry is healthy and balanced.

- I go through my monthly menstrual cycle with ease and comfort.

- My menstrual flow self-regulates. I have a moderate, comfortable menstrual flow.

- I never spot between menstrual cycles.

- I am free of blood clots.

- My menstrual cycle comes at the right time each month. I have a regular cycle.

- My vaginal muscles, cervix, and uterus are relaxed and comfortable.

- My uterus is normal size and shape.

- My menstrual flow leaves my body easily and effortlessly each month.

- My body feels wonderful as I start each monthly period.

- I barely know that my body is getting ready to menstruate.

- I feel wonderful each month before I menstruate.

- My ovaries and uterus are healthy.

- My thyroid gland is healthy and helps regulate my menstrual flow.

- My low back muscles feel supple and pliable with each menstrual cycle.

- I am relaxed and at ease as my period approaches.

- I desire a well-balanced and healthful diet.

- I eat only the foods that are good for my female body.

- It is a real pleasure to take good care of my body.

- I do the level of exercise that keeps my body healthy and supple.

- I handle stress easily and in a relaxed manner.

- I love my body; I feel at ease in my body.

- I create perfect health and well-being within my body.

Exercise 7: Visualizations for Premenopause

Visualization exercises help you create the mental blueprint for a healthier body. This powerful technique can stimulate the positive chemical and hormonal changes in your body, helping achieve the desired outcome. Through positive visualization, you are imaging your body the way you want it to function and to be. The body can modify its chemical and hormonal output in response to this technique and move toward a state of improved health. As a result, you may find this technique useful for reducing the symptoms that occur during the premenopause time.

Women (and men) with many types of illnesses have used visualization to their benefit. Visualization was pioneered by Carl Simonton, M.D., a cancer radiation therapist, who used this technique with his patients. Instead of seeing their cancer as a "big destructive monster," he had his patients see their immune system as big white knights or white sharks attacking the small and insignificant cancer cells and destroying them (instead of the other way around). In a substantial number of cases, he saw his patient's health improve. In this visualization exercise, I utilize an "erasure" image that helps you see any fibroids, ovarian cysts, old scar tissue, or other accumulated "wear and tear" on your body melt away and disappear. Then, these stressed areas are replaced by positive visualizations consistent with reproductive health and well-being. Skip any parts of the exercise that do not pertain to you.

- Sit in a comfortable position.

- Close your eyes. Begin to breathe deeply, slowly inhaling through your nose and exhaling through your mouth. Feel your body begin to relax.

- Imagine that you can look, as if through a magic mirror, deep inside your body.

- First, focus on any areas of your reproductive tract that you sense contain areas of damage or scarring. These can include tissue damage from old infections or areas of endometriosis.

- Next, imagine a large eraser—the kind used to erase chalk marks—entering into your pelvic area. See this eraser rubbing out areas of tissue damage or old scar tissue. See these areas begin to loosen, shrink, and finally disappear.

- Then look at your female organs. See your uterus: it is an attractive pink color. Your uterus is relaxed and supple. Any fibroid tumors are melting away as you look at them. Your uterus is becoming its normal size and shape. Your uterus has good blood circulation.

- Now, see the lining of your uterus. It is a lush, blood-rich cushion of tissue.

- Imagine that your uterus is currently in the state that occurs immediately before your menstrual cycle begins. The blood vessels in the lining of the uterus begin to constrict. See them become coiled and narrow. Visualize them as they begin to release the perfect amount of blood from the uterine lining.

- The blood flows out of the uterus in a moderate, regular flow. See the blood leave the uterus in a steady, healthy manner.

- See the uterine lining slough off into the blood flow so the uterus can prepare for the next month's cycle.

- Visualize your ovaries and fallopian tubes as they connect into the sides of the uterus. Your ovaries are shaped like almonds. See any cysts on the ovaries melt away until they disappear. Your ovaries are shiny, pink, and healthy looking. See them put out healthy levels of your female hormones, estrogen and progesterone. Your ovaries are perfectly regulated and function well each month.

- Look at your abdominal and low back muscles. They are soft and pliable with a healthy muscle tone. They are relaxed and free of tension during your menstrual period. Your abdomen is flat and your fluid balance is perfect in your pelvic area.

- Look at your entire body and enjoy the sense of peace and calm running through your body. You feel wonderful.

- Now stop visualizing the scene and go back to deep breathing.

- Open your eyes and feel very good. Visualizing these scenes should take several minutes. Be sure to linger on any images that particularly please you.

Stress Reduction Exercises for Menopause

While the physical and emotional symptoms of menopause are primarily due to the rapid and sustained drop in the estrogen and progesterone levels, stress can also play a significant role in both triggering and intensifying menopause symptoms. For example, hot flashes, the most common symptom of menopause, frequently occur when women are engaged in an activity or situation about which they feel emotionally tense or nervous. Many of my patients report an increase in the frequency of hot flashes when they have to give a speech, do a presentation in front of a group, mix at large social gatherings, or complete an important task on a tight time schedule. Thus, how well you manage stress can have tremendous repercussions on the ease or severity of your menopause symptoms. Positive beliefs and visualizations about your body during this time can decrease the level of stress hormones, thereby promoting healthier chemical and physiological responses on the body. This will help reduce the intensity of menopause-related symptoms.

In this section, I have included relaxation exercises to help you master your level of stress more effectively as a means of reducing menopausal symptoms. Other exercises have been included to help you develop a positive body image during this time of great change, in effect; using your mind to create the healthy body you would like to have during your menopausal and postmenopausal years.

Exercise 8: Meditation

Meditation requires you to sit quietly and engage in a simple and repetitive activity. By emptying your mind, you give yourself a rest. The metabolism of your body slows down. Meditating gives your mind a break from tension and worry. It is a useful exercise to do during early menopause, when every little stress is magnified by the drop in hormone levels that your body is experiencing. After meditating, you may find your mood greatly improved and your ability to handle everyday stress enhanced. This quieting of the body and mind can be very helpful to menopausal women who find their symptoms intensified by even little day-to-day stresses.

- Sit or lie in a comfortable position.

- Close your eyes and breathe deeply. Let your breathing be slow and relaxed.

- Focus all your attention on your breathing. Notice the movement of your chest and abdomen, in and out.

- Block out all other thoughts, feelings, and sensations. If you feel your attention wandering, bring it back to your breathing.

- As you inhale, say the word "peace" to yourself; as you exhale, say the word "relax" Draw out the pronunciation of the word so that it lasts for the entire breath. The word "peace" sounds like p-e-e-a-a-a-c-c-c-e-e-e. The word "relax" sounds like r-r-r-e-e-e-l-l-l-a-a-x-x. Repeating these words as you breathe will help you concentrate.

- Repeat this exercise until you feel calm and restful.

Exercise 9: Healing Meditation

This exercise induces a sense of peace and calm through a series of positive images. I have included a series of beautiful and peaceful images that will help create a positive mental state during times when life simply seems too frantic or busy. This meditation allows you to withdraw from your usual environment by going within yourself to find a place of healing. When you return, you will feel refreshed, better able to meet the daily life challenges many midlife women often deal with in addition to the physical stress of menopause.

This meditation is based on the fact that our mind and body are inextricably linked. When we visualize a beautiful scene where our body is being healed, we stimulate positive chemical and hormonal changes that can reduce pain, discomfort and irritability. Likewise, if you visualize a negative scene such as a fight with a spouse or a boss, the negative mental picture can trigger a chemical output in your body that exaggerates menopause related symptoms. The axiom "you are what you think" is quite true. I have seen the power of positive thinking, and I advise my patients that healing the body is much harder if the mind is full of angry or fearful images. Healing meditations, when practiced on a regular basis, can be a powerful healing tool. If you enjoy this form of meditation, try designing your own exercises with images that make you feel good.

- Lie on your back in a comfortable position. Inhale through your nose and exhale slowly and deeply through your mouth.

- Visualize a beautiful green meadow full of lovely fragrant flowers. In the middle of this meadow is a golden temple. See the temple emanating peace and healing.

- Visualize yourself entering this temple. You are the only person inside. It is still and peaceful. As you stand inside, you feel a healing energy fill every pore of your body with a warm, golden light. Every cell in your body that is in need of repair and healing is nourished by this light. This energy feels like a healing balm that relaxes you totally. All stress dissolves and fades from your mind. You feel totally at ease. Remain in this temple for as long as you wish.

- When you are ready to leave, open your eyes and continue your slow, deep breathing for a few more cycles.

The next two exercises will help you gain mastery over stress by learning to shrink it or even erase it with your mind. Stress is then put in a much more manageable and realistic perspective. These two exercises will also help engender a sense of power and mastery, thereby reducing nervous tension and restoring a sense of calm.

Often situations and beliefs look large and insurmountable, making us feel nervous and tense. In this scenario, women tend to feel tiny and helpless while the people or situations generating the stress appear huge and problems seem unsolvable. These feelings are often intensified during menopause when decline in hormonal levels makes our coping ability more tenuous. Situations that wouldn't normally cause women distress can create irritability, tearfulness, and a variety of other emotional responses. Some women even create mental pictures that produce feelings of helplessness.

Exercise 10: Shrinking Stress

- Sit or lie in a comfortable position. Breathe slowly and deeply.

- Visualize a situation, person or even a belief ("I can't handle more tension with my boss" or "I don't want to give that public speech") that makes you feel upset or tense.

- As you do this, you might see a person's face, a place where you're uncomfortable or simply a dark cloud. Where do you see this stressful picture? Is it above you, to one side, or in front of you? How does it look? Is it large or small, dark or light? Does it have certain colors?

- Now, slowly begin to shrink the stressful picture. Continue to see the stressful picture shrinking until it is so small that it can be held in your hands. As you hold your hand out in front of you, place the picture in the palm of your hand.

- If the stressor has a characteristic sound (such as a voice or traffic noise), hear it becoming softer. As it continues to diminish, the voice or sound becomes almost inaudible.

- Now the stressful picture is so small it can fit on the tip of a finger. Watch it shrink from there until it finally turns into a little dot and disappears.

- Often this exercise causes feelings of amusement, as well as relaxation, as the feared stressor shrinks, becomes less intimidating, and finally disappears.

Exercise 11: Erasing Stress

- Sit or lie in a comfortable position. Breathe slowly and deeply.

- Visualize a situation, person or even a belief ("I'm worried about losing my job" or "I'm uncomfortable mixing with other people at parties") that causes you to feel upset or tense.

- As you do this you might see a specific person, a place, or simply shapes and colors. Where do you see this stressful picture? Is it below you, to the side, in front of you? How does it look? Is it large or small, dark or light, or does it have a specific color?

- Imagine that a large eraser—the kind used to erase chalk marks—has floated into your hand. Actually feel and see the eraser in your hand. Take the eraser and begin to rub it over the area where the stressful picture is located. As the eraser rubs out the stressful picture, the picture begins to fade, shrink, and finally disappear. When you can no longer see the stressful picture, simply continue to focus on your deep breathing for another minute, inhaling and exhaling slowly and deeply.

Exercise 12: Glandular Breathing

Optimal endocrine function is very important for the reduction and prevention of menopausal symptoms. Healthy endocrine function is also needed for disease resistance, vitality, and energy. During menopause, the decline in output of the female hormones estrogen and progesterone is less severe when the glands regulating the hormones are healthy. In fact, small amounts of female hormones continue to be secreted from the ovaries, adrenals, and fat tissue even after menopause.

This exercise helps stimulate and energize your endocrine glands through the use of color breathing. When you direct your breath into the endocrine glands and visualize them being infused by color, the glands are stimulated in a beneficial way. The use of color breathing expands the glands' electromagnetic field. In this exercise, the color red is used. Research studies with red light have shown that this color stimulates both endocrine and immune function.

- Sit upright in a chair, your arms at your sides, palms up. Imagine a large balloon filled with red color above your head. This is a bright, vibrant tone of red that sparkles with energy. As you inhale deeply, see yourself popping this balloon and releasing the red color. Allow the red color to flow into your head and concentrate in the hypothalamus, a gland located at the base of the brain. As the hypothalamus begins to overflow with color, exhale and breathe the red out of your lungs, filling the air around you.

- As you inhale again, breathe the bright red color into your pituitary, an important endocrine gland located in your brain, right below the hypothalamus. Fill the pituitary with this color until it overflows. Then exhale deeply.

- As you continue to inhale the bright red color, let it flow into your thyroid gland, located in your neck, then into your thymus gland, located in the middle of your chest. Finally, let the color energize your adrenal glands, located in the middle of your back above the kidneys, and your ovaries, located in the pelvis. When you finish this exercise, relax for a few minutes, breathing in and out slowly and deeply.

The next two exercises present you with a series of affirmations, or positive statements, that will help you to create an excellent state of health as well as facilitate the practice of a healthy lifestyle. During the menopause years and beyond, it is not enough to exercise vigorously and follow a healthy diet; it is also important to like your body and think positive thoughts as you go through the changes related to menopause. This is because your state of health is determined by the interaction between your mind and body, by the thousands of messages you send yourself each day with your thoughts. You can aggravate your menopause symptoms with negative thoughts because when your body believes it is sick, it behaves accordingly.

You may find when repeating certain affirmations that you have negative feelings about your body and menopause; these correspond to deeply held beliefs about your body that you would like to change. This exercise is very effective in helping change negative, unhappy thoughts to positive thoughts of self-love and acceptance. Doing this exercise on a regular basis will help you like your body more as you go through the changes of menopause. You may want to emphasize certain affirmations while deleting others. Writing each affirmation three times can also be very effective.

Exercise 13: Affirmations for Menopause

- Sit in a comfortable position. Repeat the following affirmations three times.

- I go through menopause easily and effortlessly.

- My body is healthy and strong during my menopause transition.

- My body becomes healthier each day.

- My hormones are perfectly balanced and regulated.

- My body chemistry is healthy and balanced.

- My female system is strong and healthy.

- My female organs are full of health and vitality.

- My body self-regulates its temperature control effectively.

- My skin temperature feels comfortable all the time.

- I sleep well every night.

- My vagina is moist and elastic, with good circulation.

- I have sexual relations as often as I desire.

- My mood is calm and relaxed.

- I handle stress easily and effortlessly

- My breasts are healthy and full of vitality.

- My thyroid is healthy and full of vitality.

- My bones and joints are strong and healthy.

- I feel wonderful as I go through menopause.

- I love my body.

Exercise 14: Menopause Lifestyle Affirmations

- Menopause is a beautiful time of growth and change for me.

- Menopause is presenting me with many opportunities to make wonderful and positive life changes.

- I take excellent care of myself during this time of change.

- I love to nurture myself.

- I take time each day to relax and enjoy myself.

- I practice the relaxation methods that I enjoy.

- I am enjoying my life more and more. My life brings me pleasure.

- I do my work and activities in a relaxed and comfortable way.

- I enjoy the company of my family and friends. They give me pleasure.

- I eat a well-balanced and healthful diet.

- I eat the foods that keep my body strong and healthy.

- I enjoy eating the foods that are delicious and full of healthy vitamins and minerals.

- As I get older, I am becoming stronger and healthier.

- I am full of vigor and vitality.

- Each day I practice the self-help methods that I enjoy. My life is fun and exciting.

Exercise 15: Visualizations for Menopause

This exercise uses visual pictures to help you achieve a more positive body image. It can help you create a mental blueprint of how you would like your body to look and function during menopause and beyond. Positive visualizations can help your body become healthier through creating a positive system of beliefs about your health. As you see your body radiating health and vitality, you stimulate chemical changes in your body to help create this condition.

In addition, positive visualization helps modify your behavior so that you can create the body images you like. You are more likely to choose more healthful foods and nutrients as well as practice beneficial exercises and self-care techniques when you practice the visualizations.

- Close your eyes. Begin to breathe deeply. Inhale and exhale slowly. Feel your body begin to relax.

- Imagine that you can look inside your body at your vital organs.

- Look at your female organs. They are full of energy and vitality. Your ovaries, uterus, and vagina are very healthy. They have an attractive pink color. Nutrients and oxygen flow freely to them and they release their waste products from your body. Your vagina is moist, pink, and healthy. It is elastic and expandable. You are able to enjoy a healthy and active sex life.

- Look at your breasts. The tissue is smooth, without lumps or masses. They feel comfortable when you touch them.

- Look at your thyroid (the gland below your Adam's apple in your neck). It has a healthy size and texture. It regulates your metabolism perfectly and functions normally.

- Look at your bones. They are strong and sturdy. They are full of calcium and other essential nutrients.

- Now, see your face. It is smooth and relaxed. It has a smile. You feel in command of yourself. You do not feel anxious, irritable, or depressed. Your mood is wonderful. As you look at yourself in the mental mirror, you know you can handle any problems that come along competently and with ease.

- Your skin is smooth and moist. Touch your face and hands. You take wonderful care of your skin by using moisturizers, sunscreens, and limiting your sun exposure. Your skin looks lovely.

- Look at your entire body and enjoy the feeling of energy and optimism that is running through you. You are very calm and peaceful.

- Now stop visualizing the scene and return to deep breathing.

- You open your eyes and feel very good.

- Visualizing this scene should take about forty-five seconds to one minute, longer if you choose to linger with a particular image. A visualization is successful when it allows you to change your feelings about a particular situation.

How to Choose the Right Stress Reduction Exercises

This chapter has introduced you to many different ways to reduce menopause-related tension and stress and has taught you how to use mental techniques to improve your state of health. Try each exercise that pertains to your symptoms at least once. Then find the combination that works best for you. Doing the exercises you enjoy most should take no longer than 10 to 20 minutes. Ideally, do the exercises daily. Over time, they will help you handle stress better and relax more easily. They will also help you change negative thoughts and feelings about menopause into positive, self-nurturing ones.

19

Physical Exercise and Menopause

Many menopausal women neglect engaging in physical activity on a regular basis. In fact, nearly 17 percent of women are completely inactive, never exercising at all. This is unfortunate because exercise is one of the most beneficial self-help activities that a menopausal woman can do. A regular exercise program will help relieve and prevent common menopause symptoms including hot flashes, vaginal and bladder atrophy, emotional changes, and mood swings. In addition, physical activity can help prevent the longer-term problems associated with hormonal withdrawal and aging, such as bone loss, heart disease, and changes in weight and appearance. Many of the signs associated with aging actually result from physical inactivity. A sedentary lifestyle with little walking, lifting, or stretching causes poor circulation, shortness of breath, joint and muscle stiffness, fatigue and depression.

Treating Specific Menopause Symptoms with Exercise

Exercise should play a part in a good menopause self-help program. Let's examine how exercise can decrease your specific menopausal symptoms and improve your health.

Hot Flashes and Night Sweats

Women vary greatly in how they experience hot flashes in early menopause. Interestingly, the frequency and severity of hot flashes are not simply due to each woman's physiological programming (although this is certainly an important determinant). Many lifestyle factors also affect how severe the hot flash symptoms will be. Emotional stress and use of high-stress foods such as alcohol, coffee and chocolate can play an important role in triggering hot flashes. Luckily, both of these factors can be modified through good lifestyle habits. Exercise in particular can help reduce hot flashes for many women.

During their early menopausal years, many women find that they are more sensitive to everyday life stresses. Situations such as doing a presentation in front of a group, mixing with other people at social gatherings, or dealing with (or even thinking about) emotionally-charged family issues can bring on a series of hot flashes in susceptible women. Exercise practiced on a regular basis (at least three times a week for a half hour) can be the perfect remedy for discharging stress. In one study of the effect of aerobic exercise on hot flashes, 55 percent of the women reported a decrease in the severity of hot flashes. Their estrogen levels also rose following the exercise session. This link between estrogen levels and exercise emphasizes the importance of regular physical activity.

As well as elevating estrogen levels, exercise can help reduce the intensity of fight-or-flight stress response, which can be triggered by any situation that appears to be potentially dangerous or frightening. This response is mediated by the sympathetic nervous system which speeds up and heightens physiological functions we're normally unaware of, such as heart rate, skeletal muscle tension, and output of adrenal and thyroid hormones, all adjustments that allow a quick response to a threatening situation.

Unfortunately, many menopausal women may be in a state of constant nervous tension due to both the many social issues that occur during this time of change, as well as to their body's changing hormones and physiology. This can put women in a constant state of panic so they react to small stresses in the same way they would to real emergencies.

Exercise can help reduce hot flashes by providing an alternative way to discharge tension without harming your personal relationships or your body. After physical exercise, both the body and mind are calm, as physiological parameters, including breathing and heart rate, return to a more healthful resting level. The life problems and issues that trigger hot flashes often seem more manageable after a good exercise workout.

Exercise can also help reduce intake of frequently used addictive foods, alcohol and caffeine-containing coffee, tea, and chocolate, all of which can trigger hot flashes. Often those foods are over consumed as a way to handle stress or as a pick-up to boost energy. Women can consciously substitute regular exercise in place of more harmful ways of dealing with stress or low energy states, thereby reducing the frequency of their hot flashes as an added benefit. In addition, an exercise program practiced three to five times a week is a positive habit that provides many health benefits in addition to reducing hot flashes.

Vaginal and Bladder Atrophy

Vaginal and bladder changes, such as thinning of the mucosa and loss of elasticity, trouble many menopausal women. These changes can lead to soreness and irritation of the vagina, urethra, and bladder, as well as pain during intercourse. In addition, recurrent bladder and vaginal infections are common. While these problems are due primarily to the decrease in female hormones needed to stimulate healthy tissue in this area, poor blood circulation and muscle tone in the pelvic area can also contribute to vaginal and bladder symptoms. This can be helped tremendously by regular physical activity, particularly when the pelvic muscles are involved.

One of the best types of physical exercise is sexual activity, which stimulates vaginal lubrication, good blood circulation to the vagina, and rhythmic movement of the pelvic muscles. Studies have shown that women who continue to be sexually active after menopause (with at least one sexual encounter per week), either through sexual intercourse or masturbation, tend to have fewer signs of vaginal aging. There is less vaginal shrinkage and loss of elasticity because the tissue is being gently stretched on a regular basis. In addition, women who remain sexually active tend to secrete higher levels of androgens (the male hormones) from their ovaries after menopause, although estrogen levels are unaffected. Interestingly enough, it is the small amounts of androgens that women secrete, rather than estrogen, that are responsible for maintaining libido or sexual desire.

Even nonsexual touching can improve circulation to the pelvic area through massage or gentle touching of the whole body, which promotes muscle relaxation and improves circulation. Couples can give much pleasure to each other through learning simple massage techniques; single women can exchange massages with friends.

General aerobic exercise will help promote better muscle tone and blood circulation to the pelvic area. Physical exercise such as walking, tennis, or low-impact aerobics causes a vigorous pumping action of the skeletal muscles throughout the body, including the pelvis. This brings blood flow, oxygenation, and needed nutrients to the muscles in this area; it also helps remove waste products of metabolism, such as carbon dioxide and lactic acid, to maintain healthy vaginal and bladder tissues.

Local pelvic area exercises improve bladder control, vaginal elasticity, and can increase sexual pleasure. One set of exercises was developed by Dr. Arnold Kegel in the 1940s. The Kegel exercises strengthen the muscles that surround the urethra, vagina, and anus. Women who do these exercises report that they are more aware of their vagina, have more sensation in their pelvic area, and find sex more pleasurable. They also notice less leaking of urine when they cough, sneeze, or laugh, a very common symptom following menopause.

Dr. Kegel's exercises are simple and easy to do. They can be done any-where—sitting, standing, or lying down. You may want to perform these exercises at least five times a day. They have been reported to help decrease symptoms of urinary incontinence in more than 50 percent of women who practice them. They can be performed as follows:

- Draw up the vaginal muscles slowly, hold for three seconds, then relax. Repeat the process ten times.

- Then tense and relax your vaginal muscles rapidly. Repeat the process ten times.

The Kegel exercises should be performed as part of a preventive program for vaginal and bladder health for the rest of your life along with any other therapy such as the use of estrogen.

Psychological Symptoms and Insomnia

Menopause can cause significant symptoms of emotional distress such as anxiety, irritability, mood swings, and depression as well as poor sleep quality. Regular aerobic exercise improves menopause-related emotional symptoms by improving the physiology and chemistry of the brain. This promotes healthy brain function and emotional well-being. After exercising, you will feel peaceful, calmer and even happier. You will even feel more refreshed and energized. How does exercise promote such significant emotional changes? Exercise brings better oxygenation and circulation to the brain and nerves. By opening up and dilating blood vessels of the head and brain, more nutrients flow to, and waste products are removed from, this vital system. In fact, 20 percent of the blood flow from the heart goes directly to the brain. The brain also utilizes a large share (about 20 percent) of the body's nutrients and energy.

Research studies of adults who exercise compared with similar adults who are sedentary show striking differences in a variety of mental functions. Adults engaged in an active exercise program have better concentration, clearer and quicker thinking, and better problem solving capabilities. After undertaking a regular exercise program, reaction time and short-term memory improved. This can be an important preventive benefit for women past midlife who want to preserve peak intellectual and mental capacity for the rest of their lives.

Not only does regular exercise induce functional improvements in the brain, it alters brain chemistry through the increased production of beta endorphins. Beta endorphins, chemicals released from the pituitary glands, act as natural opiates produced by the body. They are chemically similar to the pain reliever morphine but are two hundred times more potent. Endorphins have a dramatic effect on mood. When levels in the body are high, they improve a woman's general sense of well-being.

Research studies demonstrate that brisk aerobic exercise such as running can increase beta endorphin levels as much as fivefold. Measurements taken a half hour after the end of an exercise session showed that beta endorphin levels were still higher than starting levels. Beta endorphins are thought to be responsible for the "runner's high" that marathon runners experience. Some women who exercise regularly report feelings of elation, euphoria, and even bliss.

Because beta endorphins elevate mood and promote well-being, exercise can also be an effective antidote for depression. While the standard treatment for depression is psychotherapy and antidepressant medication, a number of interesting chemical studies have shown that exercise helps relieve moderate depression in a significant fashion. This can be true in women of all ages, benefiting young women as well as women in their menopause years. One interesting study, done at the University of Virginia, studied depressed college students. During the study period, students who jogged regularly showed significant reduction in depression symptoms, while those students who did not exercise had virtually no change in their symptoms. This finding has significance for menopausal women when emotional symptoms of anxiety coexist with depression. Menopausal women often complain that their moods vacillate; for these women, exercise can be a powerful antidote, balancing and calming emotional upsets of all types.

Menopausal women often have difficulty sleeping at night. While hot flashes may initially awaken women in the middle of the night, falling back to sleep may be difficult. Some women find that once they are awake, their mind becomes active and may stay busy with "chatter" and self-talk for two to three hours.

Some women try strong sleeping medications or alcoholic beverages to induce sleep. In extreme cases, this can lead to drug and alcohol abuse as women increase their intake in an effort to sleep so they are not constantly exhausted from sleep deprivation during the day.

Exercise can also reduce insomnia by working off nervous energy and diffusing the fight-or-flight response to stress. After exercise, both the body and mind are calmer with the physiological parameters such as breathing and heart rate returning to a more healthful resting level. Regular exercise may also contribute to reducing alcohol and drug dependence. However, brisk exercise should not be done late in the day by women suffering from menopause-related insomnia because the energizing effects of the exercise are not desirable late at night. It is better to exercise earlier in the day if sleep induction is one of your main goals.

In summary, vigorous exercise brings blood to the brain as well as the endocrine glands and female reproductive tract. It can have a tremendously beneficial effect on mood, balancing and calming the emotions by helping promote healthier brain and nerve function. Anxiety, depression, and insomnia can be combated by a regular exercise program.

Osteoporosis

One of the most important reasons for engaging in regular physical activity during menopause is the prevention of osteoporosis. While the use of estrogen and nutrients, such as calcium and vitamin D, are necessary for building healthy bones and preventing loss of bone mass, they are not enough by themselves to prevent osteoporosis if a woman neglects physical activity and lives a sedentary life.

Bones demand exercise for their healthy maintenance. Lack of exercise will cause bone and muscle mass loss. This is true even in otherwise healthy, low-risk groups. For example, young people who are confined to bed for an illness lose bone mass.

While all aerobic exercise will strengthen your cardiovascular system and keep your muscles fit and toned, it will not necessarily preserve bone mass. To prevent osteoporosis, exercise must focus on the long bones of the body and make them work against the force of gravity. As a result, walking, trampolining, and dancing are excellent osteoporosis prevention exercises for the lower body. For the upper body, racket sports, weight lifting (with light weights), and tennis all help prevent bone loss in the torso and arms. An added benefit from participating in these activities is an increase in muscle mass and strength. In contrast, swimming will not help to preserve bone mass because water neutralizes the effect of gravity on the body. (Water activities, however, are excellent for women with muscular and joint problems, because they enhance flexibility and reduce stiffness.)

For best results, weight-bearing exercise must be practiced on a regular basis and in a sustained fashion. At least 30 minutes per session, three times a week should be done for bone protection. In fact, one study in *The New England Journal of Medicine* reported that women who exercised three times a week and used calcium supplements lost significantly less bone mass (about one percent) over a two-year time period. However, women in the same study who did more than the recommended amount of exercise (the equivalent of two hours per day of brisk walking), lost no bone mass at all.

Unfortunately, many women over the ages of 45 to 50 are too inactive for adequate osteoporosis prevention. Many women have desk jobs requiring them to sit all day and there is little time to exercise. Other women choose not to exercise because they are self-conscious about their body shape or weight (which becomes more difficult to maintain with increasing age) or because their energy levels are diminished. In all of these cases, it is important to resist the urge to be sedentary. Keep moving and institute a regular exercise program combining both weight bearing and aerobic conditioning. Even short sessions of activity can make a difference.

Heart Disease

Heart disease is the biggest killer of women in the postmenopausal years; the incidence of heart disease increases tenfold in women between the ages of 55 and 65. Statistics such as these are unnecessary because heart disease can be prevented. The actual risk of developing heart disease, even if it is prevalent in your family, can be greatly lowered by practicing a healthy lifestyle. Reducing fat intake and emotional stress along with a regular program of aerobic exercise are important components of an effective heart disease prevention program.

Aerobic Exercise Benefits the Heart

Exercise conditions the heart and lungs to work more efficiently. A healthy heart is a well-functioning pump. It beats slowly and forcefully, circulating blood throughout the body with each stroke. Once an exercise program is initiated, the resting heart rate slows down quite rapidly. Research studies show that the beneficial changes can occur quickly, often within several months.

A healthier heart also reacts less dramatically during periods of stress. When nervous tension causes the adrenal glands to pump out stressor hormones, a conditioned heart will not experience a significant rise in heart rate. In a stressful situation, a fit person may have only a slight rise in heart rate, while a sedentary person may experience a terrifying pounding of the heart and shortness of breath. Not only does a fit person tend to stay calm and more in control of emotions during a difficult situation, but in periods of extreme stress, good physical conditioning may help prevent a heart attack.

Lungs function more efficiently with exercise, too. They expand more fully and fill with oxygen. Exercise helps dilate and expand the network of blood vessels in the body, so more blood reaches the muscles and vital organ systems. The effects of exercise will help prevent blood clotting and lower the level of fat in the blood vessels. A healthy heart and lungs mean greater endurance and physical energy. You can go through your daily activities more easily, with a sense of vigor and well-being.

Women who have been sedentary for a long period of time should not suddenly begin a vigorous program of aerobic activity. Starting a cardio-vascular fitness program should be done gradually, and before beginning, I strongly recommend that you see your physician for a cardiovascular risk assessment. This is particularly important if you have a previous history of cardiovascular disease, diabetes mellitus, or high blood pressure. Your physician can identify any potential problems and help you tailor your exercise program.

Weight Control and Appearance

Exercise is an absolute necessity for most menopausal women for weight control and body tone. As our endocrine glands change with age, we tend to digest and metabolize food less efficiently. Pounds accumulate rapidly after menopause, as our bodies need fewer calories for maintenance. Some of my patients complained that they gained 10 to 15 pounds after menopause. These pounds can be very difficult to lose no matter how hard they diet. Many women eat smaller and smaller meals to maintain their weight. Older women who want to maintain their appearance are often in a state of chronic dieting to prevent "middle-age spread."

Luckily, exercise can provide midlife women with an antidote to unwanted pounds. Rather than cutting down caloric intake to starvation levels, increase your level of physical activity. Exercise allows you to maintain your weight far more easily than dieting because it burns calories and stimulates your metabolism. A regular aerobic program of walking, dancing, swimming, or other activity is a must to control your weight and allow you to look and feel your best. A regular exercise program also aids your appearance by helping preserve attractive body contours, toning muscles and improving skin condition. Exercise increases blood circulation to the skin, keeping the skin pink, soft, and supple. The skin of women who don't exercise frequently looks pale and unhealthy.

It is important, however, not to try to be too thin with the onset of menopause. Women who are too thin have lower estrogen levels and are at higher risk for such menopause problems as osteoporosis and hot flashes. Aim for a weight level and appearance that is attractive and not extreme—neither too thin nor obese. Set your weight and exercise program at a level that feels comfortable, is easy to maintain, and looks good.

Building a Personal Exercise Program Evaluating your Fitness Level

As you move from a sedentary lifestyle to a regular exercise program, evaluate your level of fitness. It is important to know if you have any undiagnosed medical problems that could impact your proper level of activity. This includes problems such as thyroid disease, hypertension, and blood sugar imbalances commonly found in menopausal women. A complete medical examination is important for a menopausal woman beginning an exercise program after a long period of being sedentary.

Your physician should check your heart, lungs, pulse rate, and other physical parameters to evaluate your exercise fitness. In addition, blood and urine tests are frequently ordered. These tests can vary, based on the particular symptoms you report to your physician as well as the examination itself. Depending on your age and symptoms, a general chemistry panel that checks the blood levels of minerals, as well as the health of various organs such as the thyroid, may be required. If you don't understand any terms or tests your physician uses, ask for more information. An informed and educated woman can do a much better job in planning and participating in her own wellness program. Once you have received a clean bill of health or understand any health limitations, you are ready to begin planning your exercise program.

Choosing an Exercise Program

The type of exercise regimen you choose can vary greatly depending on the goals you wish to accomplish. If your main goal is to relieve menopause-related anxiety and stress and improve your general health and well-being, then aerobic exercise is best. This is because aerobic exercise promotes cardiovascular and respiratory health, which, in turn, promotes relaxation and reduces the tendency toward menopause-related insomnia. Because it requires active work on the part of your skeletal and heart muscles, it reduces the muscle tension that often accompanies menopause-related nervous tension. Aerobic exercise includes jogging, walking, bicycle riding, skiing, swimming, dancing, jumping rope, and skating.

Women who are at high risk of osteoporosis will want to emphasize exercises that require weight-bearing stress on the long bones. Combining brisk walking with weight lifting or racquet sports can give the bones the workout they need and increase bone mass.

Women for whom sexuality is an important part of their emotional and physical well-being may find engaging in frequent sexual activity, or even massage, a pleasurable form of physical activity. For women who cannot participate in vigorous physical activity due to a pre-existing cardio-vascular condition (or lack of energy), then slower-paced activities such as golf or walking could provide a helpful degree of physical exercise as well as the benefits of socializing.

Many menopausal women notice the onset of arthritis symptoms or muscle tightness and tension during this time. As an antidote, I recommend exercises such as stretching that promote joint and muscle flexibility. Stretches are performed slowly, along with deep breathing, in a relaxed and careful manner. They are helpful in slowing down an anxious system whose physiology is set on overdrive.

Finally, gardening can promote peace of mind and relaxation along with physical activity. Pulling weeds and digging up the ground involve bending, lifting, and upper-body movements, which rapidly dissipate anxiety.

Often, women may combine two or three types of exercise activities to meet a variety of goals. Whatever form of exercise you choose, make sure it meets the goals of promoting optimal health and well-being as well as providing abundant levels of energy.

Motivating Yourself to Exercise

If you encounter mental obstacles to beginning and sticking with a regular menopause exercise program, there are many ways to overcome this resistance. Be sure you are clear why you don't want to exercise so you can address the issues directly. Keeping the exercise diary found in the workbook section should help you pinpoint areas of resistance.

- Exercise at the time of day that feels most natural. For example, if you are a late riser, don't try to exercise early in the morning. Exercise when you are the least hurried and stressed by your schedule. If your longest amount of free time is in the late afternoon between work and dinner, put aside that time to engage in physical activity.
- Exercise in an attractive setting. If you run or walk, pick a setting near you that promotes peace and calm. Walk or run in a park, on a beach, or on a quiet residential street. Avoid areas with lots of cars and traffic congestion.

- Exercise with a friend or support person. This can be a great help in motivating and encouraging you to begin and stick with an exercise program.

- Use your mind to disconnect from your daily activities. Positive mental exercises can help you relax before starting physical activity. Many women find that a few minutes of doing visualizations (seeing themselves performing and enjoying the exercise routine in their minds) or saying affirmations (making positive statements about the benefits of exercise) prepares them for their exercise routine.

- Listen to music while you exercise. Many women find that the exercise period goes by more quickly and the process is more fun and enjoyable while listening to music. Be sure to choose music that is soft and relaxing if you are doing stretching exercises. This type of music will help improve your mood and relax you further. Fast paced music is more appropriate for quick-moving sessions of aerobic exercise.

- Be sure to choose an exercise activity that you enjoy. Don't pick an activity that you find boring. Refer to the activity chart at the end of this chapter if you need help in selecting an activity that looks interesting.

Beginning an Exercise Program for Menopause

Before you begin a menopause-relief exercise program, read the following guidelines. They will help you perform your exercise in an optimally beneficial manner. These guidelines are particularly useful for women just beginning regular exercise after leading a sedentary lifestyle. Getting a good start when beginning the program can make a major difference in how well you enjoy and stick to your chosen physical activity.

- During the first week or two of your program, build up your exercise level gradually. Keep initial exercise workouts short.

- For example, you might start out exercising every other day for ten minutes. Increase the length of your sessions by five-minute increments until you are exercising between 30 and 60 minutes per session.

- Exercise in a relaxed and unhurried manner. Set aside adequate time so you do not feel rushed. Anytime you feel anxiety, panic, or excessive muscle tension, stop the exercise. Then, re-evaluate your pace to see if it is too vigorous. Initially you might want to exercise with another person who can provide support and companionship.

- Wear loose, comfortable clothing. If you are doing stretching, you may want to do the exercised without socks to give your feet complete freedom of movement and to prevent slipping.

- Evacuate your bowels and/or bladder before you begin to exercise. Try to exercise at least 90 minutes before a meal and wait at least two hours after eating to exercise. Working out before dinner is particularly good because it helps diffuse tension that has accumulated throughout the day.

- Avoid exercising when ill or extremely stressed. Instead, do the stress-reduction exercises provided in this book.

- Move slowly and carefully when starting each exercise session. This promotes muscle flexibility and helps prevent injury

- Breathe deeply and evenly when you are exercising; this will give you more endurance and you will tire less easily.

- Always rest for a few minutes after completing the exercises.

Activities for Menopausal Women

- walking
- bicycle riding
- skiing
- swimming
- aerobic dancing
- low-impact aerobics
- ice skating
- roller skating or inline skating
- tennis
- table tennis
- golf
- croquet
- bowling
- stretching
- weight lifting
- gardening

Benefits of Exercise

- Helps relieve hot flashes
- Helps relieve vaginal and bladder atrophy
- Relieves anxiety, irritability, insomnia and depression
- Helps prevent osteoporosis
- Conditions heart, lungs, and muscles
- Helps prevent heart disease
- Helps control weight and improve appearance
- Improves function of vital organs such as digestive tract and nervous system
- Improves strength, stamina and flexibility
- Increases vigor and energy

20

Stretches for Menopause

Stretches can benefit both the body and the mind, bringing energy and balance. This is particularly helpful to women who are currently in menopause or in the menopause transition because their hormonal levels and body chemistry may be fluctuating rapidly. This can leave women feeling out of balance and truly victims of their changing bodies. Stretching exercises level out this physiological instability by relaxing and gently stretching every muscle in the body, promoting better blood circulation and oxygenation to all cells and tissues. This helps optimize the function of the endocrine glands and the organs of the female reproductive tract. Stretching exercises also improve the health and well-being of the digestive tract, nervous system, and all other organ systems.

The stretching exercises included in this chapter address many specific menopause-related symptoms and issues, such as bone strength, cardiovascular and breast health, of concern to all women past midlife. You may want to begin by trying all the stretches, then practicing on a regular basis those exercises that bring you the most symptom relief and general health benefits. If you prefer, begin with the exercises that offer relief for the specific symptoms of greatest concern.

General Techniques for Stretches

When doing stretching exercises, it is important that you focus and concentrate on the positions. First, let your mind visualize how the exercise is to look, and then follow with the correct body placement in the pose. The exercises are done through slow, controlled stretching movements. This slowness allows you to have greater control over your body movements. You minimize the possibility of injury and maximize the benefit to the particular area of the body where your attention is being focused.

Pay close attention to the initial instructions. Look at the placement of the body in the photographs. This is very important, for if the pose is practiced properly, you are much more likely to have relief from your symptoms.

In summary, as you begin these exercises:

- Visualize the pose in your mind, then follow with proper placement of the body.

- Move slowly through the pose. This will help promote flexibility of the muscles and prevent injury

- Follow the breathing instructions provided in the exercise. Most important, do not hold your breath. Allow your breath to flow in and out easily and effortlessly.

Practicing stretches regularly in a slow, unhurried fashion will gradually loosen your muscles, ligaments and joints. You may be surprised at how supple you can become over time. If you experience any pain or discomfort, you have probably overreached your current ability and should immediately reduce the amount of the stretching until you can proceed without discomfort. Be careful, as muscular injuries take time to heal. If you do strain a muscle, immediately apply ice to the injured area for ten minutes. Use the ice pack two to three times a day for several days. If the pain persists, see your doctor.

If you wish more background and information on stretching, refer to the books listed in the bibliography at the end of this book.

Stretch 1

This exercise energizes the entire female reproductive tract, thyroid, liver, intestines and kidneys. It is helpful for premenopausal women with dysfunctional bleeding, as well as women with menopausal symptoms such as hot flashes, because it improves circulation and oxygenation to the pelvic region, thereby promoting healthier ovarian function. This exercise also strengthens the lower back, abdomen, buttocks, and legs, and prevents lower back pain and cramps.

Lie face down on the floor. Make fists with both your hands and place them under your hips. This prevents compression of the lumbar spine while doing the exercise.

Straighten your body and raise your right leg with an upward thrust as high as you can, keeping your hips on your fists. Hold for 5 to 20 seconds if possible.

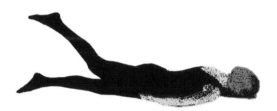

Lower the leg and slowly return to your original position. Repeat on the left side. Remember to keep your hips resting on your fists. Repeat 10 times.

Repeat 10 times with both legs together.

Stretch 2

This exercise improves blood circulation through the pelvis, thereby promoting healthier ovarian function. It helps relieve menopausal symptoms such as hot flashes and controls excessive bleeding in premenopausal women. The exercise helps calm anxiety and also strengthens the back and abdominal muscles.

Lie down and press the small of your back into the floor. This permits you to use your abdominal muscles without straining your lower back.

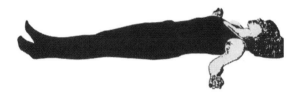

Raise your right leg slowly while breathing in. Keep your back flat on the floor and let the rest of your body remain relaxed. Move your leg very slowly; imagine your leg being pulled up smoothly by a spring. Do not move your leg in a jerky manner. Hold for a few breaths. Lower your leg and breathe out.

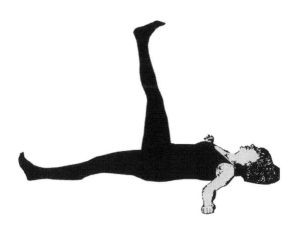

Repeat the same exercise on your left side. Then alternate legs, repeating the exercise 5 to 10 times.

Stretch 3

This exercise opens the entire pelvic region and energizes the female reproductive tract, improving ovarian function as well as normalizing excessive or irregular menstrual flow; diminution of menopausal symptoms may also occur. It is helpful for varicose veins and improves circulation in the legs.

Lie on your back with your legs against the wall and extended out in a V or an arc, and your arms extended to the side.

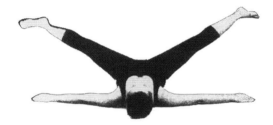

Hips should be as close to the wall as possible, buttocks on the floor. Legs should be spread apart as far as they can and still remain comfortable. Breathing easily, hold for 1 minute, allowing the inner thighs to relax.

Bring legs together and hold for 1 minute.

Stretch 4

This exercise energizes and rejuvenates the female reproductive tract and tones the abdominal organs (pancreas, liver and adrenals). It emphasizes freer pelvic movement with controlled breathing.

Lie on your back with your knees bent and your feet on the floor close to your buttocks.

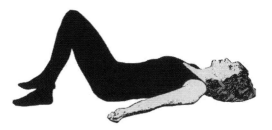

Exhale and press the lower back into the floor, raising the buttocks slightly. Arch your back slightly.

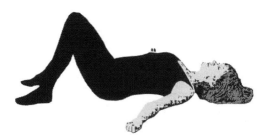

Inhale and lift your lower back off the floor. This stretches the region from the sternum to the pelvis.

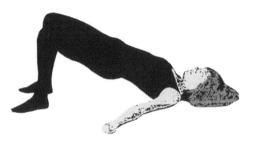

Repeat this exercise 10 times. Always lift your navel up on the in-breath. Always elongate your spine and press the lower back down on the out-breath.

Stretch 5

This is an excellent exercise for stretching the abdominal and pelvic muscles. Menopause-related vaginal and bladder symptoms are reduced by promoting better circulation and relaxation in the pelvic region. It is also helpful in reducing pelvic congestion.

Lie on your back with your knees bent. Spread your feet apart, flat on the floor.

Place your hands around your ankles, holding them firmly.

As you inhale, arch your pelvis up and hold for a few seconds. As you exhale, relax and lower your pelvis several times.

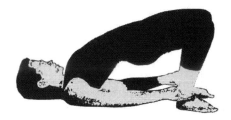

Repeat this exercise several times.

Stretch 6

This exercise helps relieve menopause-related fatigue and lack of vitality, elevating your mood and improving stamina. The exercise also stretches the entire spine and helps relieve lower back pain and cramps. It stretches the abdominal muscles and strengthens the back, hips and thighs. It also stimulates the digestive organs and endocrine glands.

Lie face down on the floor, arms at your sides.

Slowly bend your legs at the knees and bring your feet up toward your buttocks.

Reach back with your arms and carefully take hold of first one foot and then the other. Flex your feet to make grasping them easier.

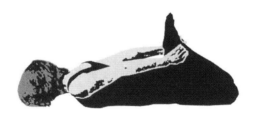

Inhale and raise your trunk from the floor as far as possible and lift your head. Bring your knees as close together as possible.

Squeeze the buttocks while raising them off the floor. Imagine your body looking like a gently curved bow. Hold for 10 to 15 seconds.

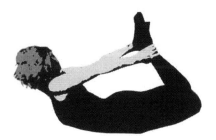

Slowly release the posture. Allow your chin to touch the floor and finally release your feet and return them slowly to the floor. Return to your original position. Repeat 5 times.

Stretch 7

Excellent for calming anxiety and stress due to emotional causes, this exercise will also relieve menopause-related anxiety and irritability. The exercise gently stretches the lower back and is one of the most effective exercises for relieving menstrual cramps and low back pain.

Sit on your heels. Bring your forehead to the floor, stretching the spine as far over your head as possible. Close your eyes.

Hold for as long as comfortable.

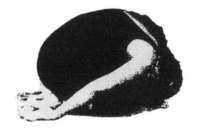

Stretch 8

This exercise relieves anxiety and stress due to emotional causes or menopause-related anxiety and tension. It relieves menstrual cramps and low back pain as well as reducing eye tension and swelling in the face.

Lie on your back with a rolled towel placed under your knees. Your arms should be at your sides, palms up.

Close your eyes and relax your whole body. Inhale slowly, breathing from the diaphragm. As you inhale, visualize the energy in the air around you being dawn in through your entire body. Imagine your body is porous and open like a sponge, drawing in this energy and revitalizing every cell of your body.

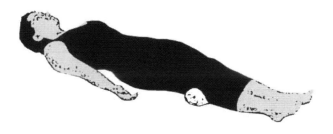

Exhale slowly and deeply, allowing all tension to drain from your body.

Stretch 9

This pose reduces anxiety and nervous tension and will help eliminate tension headaches and insomnia. It improves flexibility of the spine, reducing stiffness and back pain.

Lie on your back with your legs bent and your feet together. Place your hands on the sides of both ankles to keep your legs together.

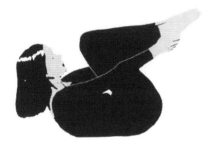

As you inhale, raise your legs up over your head. Make sure that the posture is comfortable by adjusting the angle of your legs. To do this, bend your knees to apply pressure between the shoulder blades.

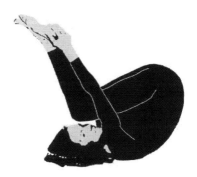

Hold this posture for one minute, breathing slowly and deeply.

Return to the original position, lying flat on your back with your eyes closed. Relax in this position for several minutes.

Stretch 10

If your goal is to strengthen bone mass by increasing weight bearing on the legs, hips and spine, this exercise will help you accomplish increasing bone mass. It also improves balance and posture.

Standing erect, focus your eyes on a stationary point. Place one foot against the opposite thigh, so that one leg is bearing your weight.

Slowly raise your arms over your head. Hold for a count of 5.

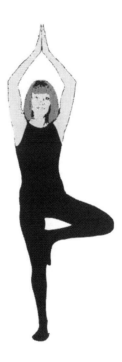

Reverse sides. Repeat 3 times.

Note: You may place one hand on the wall for support if needed.

Stretch 11

This exercise increases circulation to the upper half of the body, energizing and stimulating the body. It also loosens and stretches tense muscles in the upper body, especially the shoulder and back, and expands the lungs.

Stand easily. Arms should be at your sides; feet are hip distance apart.

Extend your arms forward until your palms touch.

Bring your arms slowly and gracefully back until you can clasp them behind your back.

Exhale, then straighten your clasped hands and arms as far as you can without discomfort. Remember to stand upright; body should not bend forward. Breathe deeply into chest.

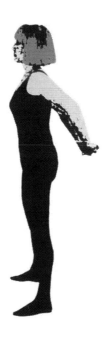

Inhale deeply and bend backward from the waist. Keep your hands clasped and your arms held high.

Drop your head backward a few inches and look upward as you relax your shoulders and the back of your neck.

Hold this position for a few seconds.

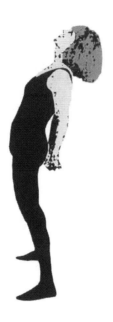

As you hold your breath, bend forward at the waist, bringing your clasped hands and arms up over your back.

Relax your neck muscles and keep your knees straight. Hold for a few seconds.

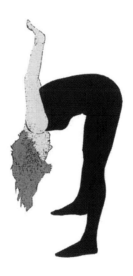

Exhale as you return to the upright position. Unclasp your hands and allow your arms to rest easily at your sides.

Repeat entire sequence 3 times.

Choosing the Right Stretch Technique

From among the many specific stretching poses in this chapter, you can choose the best exercises to provide relief for your personal menopausal symptoms by using the accompanying chart. Try all the poses that pertain to your specific symptoms to see which ones bring you the most relief and practice those poses on a regular basis along with your exercise program. The combination of stretches plus a good aerobic and strength-building program should help relieve and delay menopause-related symptoms and improve your general state of health.

Symptoms	*Exercise*
Entire female reproductive tract	Stretch 1, Stretch 2, Stretch 3, Stretch 4, Stretch 5, Stretch 6
Excessive or irregular menstrual bleeding	Stretch 1, Stretch 2, Stretch 3
Hot flashes	Stretch 1, Stretch 2, Stretch 3, Stretch 4, Stretch 5, Stretch 6
Insomnia	Stretch 7, Stretch 8, Stretch 9
Psychological symptoms—anxiety depression, fatigue	Stretch 6, Stretch 7, Stretch 8, Stretch 9
Vaginal atrophy and bladder symptoms	Stretch 1, Stretch 2, Stretch 3, Stretch 4, Stretch 5, Stretch 6
Osteoporosis	Stretch 10
Cardiovascular health	Stretch 11
Breast health	Stretch 11

21

Acupressure for Menopause

Acupressure is a traditional Asian healing technique of applying finger pressure to specific points on the body to help treat and prevent symptoms of various ailments. Over the years, many of my menopause patients have tried acupressure and it really works! Acupuncture, where the points are stimulated by needles, is done by a trained professional. While acupressure is not a cure-all, many women have reported significant relief from such common menopausal symptoms as hot flashes, fatigue, insomnia and mood swings.

How Does Acupressure Work?

When specific acupressure points are pressed, they create changes on two levels. On the physical level, acupressure affects muscular tension, blood circulation, and other physiological parameters. On a more subtle level, traditional Asian healing believes that acupressure also builds the body's life energy to promote healing. Acupressure is based on the belief of a life energy in the body called chi. It is different from, yet similar to, electromagnetic energy. Health is a state in which the chi is present in sufficient amounts and is equally distributed throughout the body energizing all the cells and tissues of the body.

The life energy runs through the body in channels called meridians. When working in a healthy manner, these channels distribute the energy evenly throughout the body, sometimes on the surface of the skin and, at times, deep inside the body in the organs. Disease occurs when the energy flow in a meridian is blocked or stopped. As a result, the internal organs that correspond to the meridians can show symptoms of disease. The meridian flow can be corrected by stimulating the points on the skin surface. These points can be treated easily by acupressure. When the normal flow of energy through the body is resumed, the body can then heal itself spontaneously.

You or a friend can stimulate the acupressure points through safe and painless finger pressure by following simple instructions.

How to Perform Acupressure

Acupressure should be done when you are relaxed. The room should be warm and quiet. Make sure your hands are clean and nails trimmed (to avoid bruising). If your hands are cold, rinse them under warm water.

Work on the side of the body that has the most discomfort. If both sides are equally uncomfortable, choose either side. Just working on one side will relieve the symptoms on both sides. Energy or information seems to transfer from one side to the other.

Look carefully at the illustration for the exercise. Hold each point indicated in the exercise with a steady pressure for one to three minutes, applying pressure slowly with the tips or balls of the fingers. It is best to place several fingers over the area of the point. If you feel resistance or tension in the area where you are applying pressure, you may want to increase the pressure slightly. Make sure your hand is comfortable; if your hand starts to feel tense or tired, release the pressure a bit. The acupressure point may feel tender; this means the energy pathway or meridian is blocked.

During the treatment, the tenderness in the point should slowly fade. You may also have a sense of energy radiating from this point into the body. Many women describe this sensation as very pleasant. Don't worry if you don't feel it—not everyone does. The main goal is relief from your symptoms.

Breathe gently while doing each exercise. The photograph accompanying the exercise will help you visualize the point you will hold. All of these points correspond to specific points on the acupressure meridians. You may apply acupressure to the points once a day, or more if you continue to have symptoms.

Acupressure Exercises

Exercise 1: Balances the Entire Reproductive System

This exercise balances the energy of the female reproductive tract and is a useful exercise to begin your acupressure program. It also helps relieve low back pain and abdominal discomfort.

Equipment: This exercise uses a knotted hand towel to put pressure on hard to reach areas of the back. Place the knotted towel on these points while your two hands are on other points. This increases your ability to unblock the energy pathways of your body.

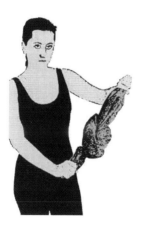 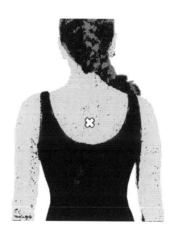

Lie on the floor with your knees up. As you lie down, place the towel between the shoulder blades on your spine. Hold each step 1 to 3 minutes.

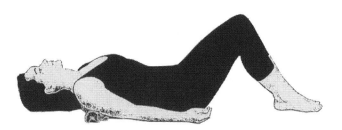

Cross your arms on your chest. Press your thumbs against the right and left inside upper arms.

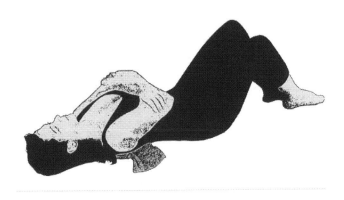

Left hand holds point at the base of the sternum (breastbone).

Right hand holds point at the base of the head (at the junction of the spine and the skull).

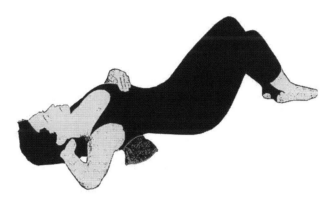

Interlace your fingers. Place them below your breasts. Fingertips should press directly against the body.

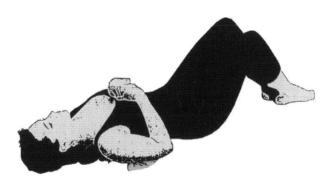

Move the knotted towel along the spine to the waistline.

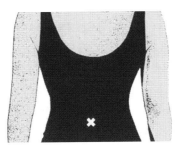

Left hand should be placed at the top of the pubic bone, pressing down.

Right hand holds point on tailbone.

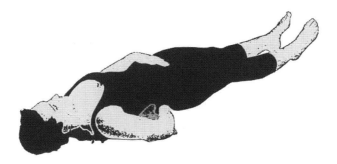

Exercise 2: Relieves Hot Flashes and Emotional Tension

This exercise helps relieve hot flashes by stimulating the entire endocrine system. It involves a very powerful point for the pituitary gland, the master regulator of the ovaries. This point also helps relax the emotional tension that many women feel during early menopause and relieves eye strain, headaches, and hay fever.

Sit upright on a chair.

Right hand holds point directly between the eyebrows, where the bridge of the nose meets the forehead. Hold the point for 1 to 3 minutes.

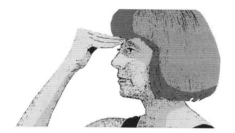

Exercise 3: Relieves Hot Flashes, Menopausal Fatigue, Anxiety, and Depression

This exercise helps relieve hot flashes as well as menopause related insomnia, depression, fatigue, and anxiety. The exercise will also relieve fatigue, anxiety, and depression women may experience prior to their menstrual periods.

Sit up and prop your back against a chair. Hold each step 1 to 3 minutes.

Right hand holds point at the base of the ball of the right foot. This point is located between the two pads of the foot.

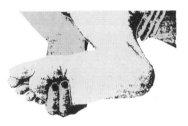

Right hand holds point in the center of your breastbone, at the level of the heart. Your fingers will fit into the indentations in this bone.

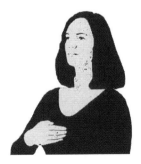

Exercise 4: Relieves Menopause-Related Insomnia

This exercise helps relieve insomnia and anxiety symptoms commonly seen in menopause. In Asian medicine, these points are called "joyful sleep" and "calm sleep".

Sit comfortably and hold these points for 1 to 3 minutes.

Left hand holds point on the inside of the right anklebone. This point is located in the indentation directly below the inner ankle bone.

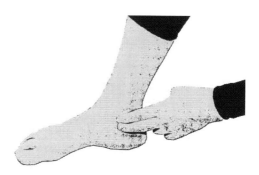

Right hand holds point located in the indentation below the right outer ankle bone.

Repeat this exercise holding the points on the left foot.

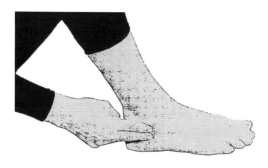

Exercise 5: Relieves Vaginal and Urinary Tract Atrophy and Promotes Healthy Bones

This exercise helps relieve symptoms of vaginal dryness and insufficient vaginal lubrication seen in menopausal women with inadequate estrogen stimulation of the vaginal tissues. These points are also used to promote strong and healthy bones. The second step in this sequence helps promote bladder health during menopause.

Sit up and prop your back against a chair. Hold each step 1 to 3 minutes.

Right hand holds point at the base of the ball of the right foot. This point is located between the two pads of the foot.

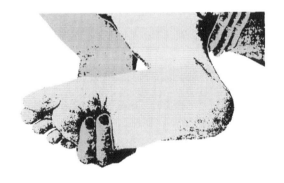

Left hand holds the point midway between the inside of the right anklebone and the Achilles tendon. The Achilles tendon is located at the back of the ankle.

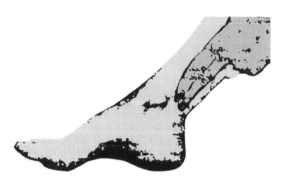

Move left hand 1 inch above the waist on the muscle to the side of the spine. Right hand holds the point on the outside of the foot, just behind the little toe.

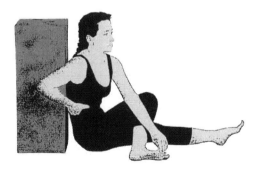

Exercise 6: Improves Cardiovascular Health

This exercise strengthens the cardiovascular system. Health problems involving this system are the major cause of death in postmenopausal women.

Sit or stand in a comfortable position. Hold each step for 1 to 3 minutes.

Right hand holds point at the base of the armpit on the chest.

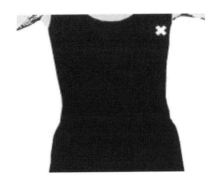

Right hand holds point at base of left wrist below the little finger.

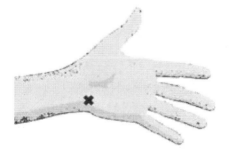

Right hand holds point in the center of your breast bone, at the level of the heart. Your fingers will fit into the indentations in this bone.

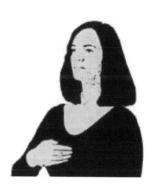

Exercise 7: Improves Breast Health

This point improves breast health by stimulating the pituitary, the master gland that regulates the output of hormones affecting the health of the breast tissue.

Sit upright in a chair or stand up. Hold each step for 1 to 3 minutes.

Right hand holds point directly between the eyebrows where the bridge of the nose meets the forehead.

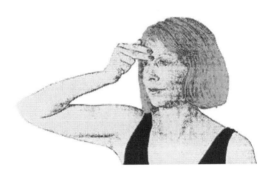

Right hand holds point on right side of chest directly above the breasts in line with the nipples. Point is between the third and fourth ribs.

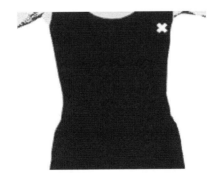

Choosing the Right Exercises

You can use the chart to select acupressure exercises most useful for your specific symptoms. Initially, try all those that pertain to your symptoms. You may find that certain ones make you feel better than others. Practice the acupressure points that bring you the most relief.

Symptoms	Acupressure Exercise
Entire female reproductive tract	1
Hot flashes	3, 4
Insomnia	4, 5
Psychological symptoms — anxiety, depression, fatigue	3, 4
Vaginal atrophy	6
Bladder symptoms	6
Osteoporosis	6
Cardiovascular health	7
Breast health	8

About Susan M. Lark, M.D.

Dr. Susan Lark is one of the foremost authorities in the fields of women's health care and alternative medicine. Dr. Lark has successfully treated many thousands of women emphasizing holistic health and complementary medicine in her clinical practice. Her mission is to provide women with unique, safe and effective alternative therapies to greatly enhance their health and well-being.

A graduate of Northwestern University Feinberg School of Medicine, she has served on the clinical faculty of Stanford University Medical School, and taught in their Division of Family and Community Medicine.

Dr. Lark is a distinguished clinician, author, lecturer and innovative product developer. Through her extensive clinical experience, she has been an innovator in the use of self-care treatments such as diet, nutrition, exercise and stress management techniques in the field of women's health, and has lectured extensively throughout the United States on topics in preventive medicine. She is the author of many best-selling books on women's health. Her signature line of nutritional supplements and skin care products are available through healthydirections.com.

One of the most widely referenced physicians on the Internet, Dr. Lark has appeared on numerous radio and television shows, and has been featured in magazines and newspapers including: Real Simple, Reader's Digest, McCall's, Better Homes & Gardens, New Woman, Mademoiselle, Harper's Bazaar, Redbook, Family Circle, Seventeen, Shape, Great Life, The New York Times, The Chicago Tribune, and The San Francisco Chronicle.

She has also served as a consultant to major corporations, including the Kellogg Company and Weider Nutrition International, and was spokesperson for The Gillette Company Women's Cancer Connection.

Dr. Lark can be contacted at (650) 561-9978 to make an appointment for a consultation.

We would enjoy hearing from you! Please share your success stories, requests for new topics and comments with us. Our team at Womens Wellness Publishing may be contacted at yourstory@wwpublishing.com. We invite you to visit our website for Dr. Lark's newest books at womenswellnesspublishing.com.

Dr. Susan's Solutions
Health Library For Women

The following books are available from Amazon.com, Amazon Kindle, iTunes, Womens Wellness Publishing and other major booksellers. Dr. Susan is frequently adding new books to her health library.

Women's Health Issues

Dr. Susan's Solutions: Healthy Heart and Blood Pressure

Dr. Susan's Solutions: Healthy Menopause

Dr. Susan's Solutions: The Anemia Cure

Dr. Susan's Solutions: The Bladder Infection Cure

Dr. Susan's Solutions: The Candida-Yeast Infection Cure

Dr. Susan's Solutions: The Chronic Fatigue Cure

Dr. Susan's Solutions: The Cold and Flu Cure

Dr. Susan's Solutions: The Endometriosis Cure

Dr. Susan's Solutions: The Fibroid Tumor Cure

Dr. Susan's Solutions: The Irregular Menstruation Cure

Dr. Susan's Solutions: The Menstrual Cramp Cure

Dr. Susan's Solutions: The PMS Cure

Emotional and Spiritual Balance

Breathing Meditations for Healing, Peace and Joy

Dr. Susan's Solutions: The Anxiety and Stress Cure

Women's Hormones

DHEA: The Fountain of Youth Hormone

Healthy, Natural Estrogens for Menopause

Pregnenolone: Your #1 Sex Hormone

Progesterone: The Superstar of Hormone Balance

Testosterone: The Hormone for Strong Bones, Sex Drive and Healthy Menopause

Diet and Nutrition

Dr. Susan Lark's Healing Herbs for Women

Dr. Susan Lark's Complete Guide to Detoxification

Enzymes: The Missing Link to Health

Healthy Diet and Nutrition for Women: The Complete Guide

Renew Yourself Through Juice Fasting and Detoxification Diets

Energy Therapies and Anti-Aging

Acupressure for Women: Relieve Symptoms of Dozens of Health Issues Through Pressure Points

Exercise and Flexibility

Stretching and Flexibility for Women

Stretching Programs for Women's Health Issues

About Womens Wellness Publishing

"Bringing Radiant Health and Wellness to Women"

Womens Wellness Publishing was founded to make a positive difference in the lives of women and their families. We are the premier publisher of print and eBooks focused on women's health and wellness. We are committed to publishing the finest quality and most comprehensive line of books that covers every area that a woman needs to create vibrant health and a joyful, fulfilling life.

Our books are written and created by the top health and wellness experts who share with you, our readers, their wisdom and extensive experience successfully treating many thousands of patients.

We encourage you to browse through our online bookstore; new books are frequently being added at womenswellnesspublishing.com. Also visit our Lifestyle Center and Customer Bonus Center for more exciting and helpful health and wellness information and resources.

Follow us on Facebook for the latest health tips, recipes, and all natural solutions to many women's health issues (facebook.com/wwpublishing).

About Our Associate Program

We invite you to become part of the Womens Wellness Publishing Community through our Associate Program. You will have the opportunity to earn generous commissions on sales that you create through your blog, social network, support groups, community groups, school & alumni groups, friends, family or other networks.

To join our program, go to our website and click "Become an Associate" (womenswellnesspublishing.com.)_We support your sales and marketing efforts by offering you and your customers:

- Free support materials with updates on all of our new book releases, promotions, and bonuses for you and your customers
- Free audio downloads, booklets, and guides
- Special discounts and sales promotions

References

Adlercreutz H, Hämäläinen E, Gorbach S, Goldin B. Dietary phyto-oestrogens and the menopause in Japan. Lancet. 1992 May 16;339(8803):1233–1233. [PubMed]

Al-Azzawi F, Palacios S. Hormonal changes during menopause. *Maturitas.* 2009;63(2):135-7.

American College of Obstetricians and Gynecologists. Herbal Products for Menopause. Patient Education Pamphlet 2003: Available at http://www.acog.org/publications/patient_education/bp158.cfm

American College of Obstetricians and Gynecologists. Use of Botanicals for Mangement of Menopausal Symptoms. Practice Bulletin 2001: 28. Available   at: http://www.acog.org/from_home/publications/misc/pb028.htm

Anderson JW, Johnstone BM, Cook-Newell ME. Meta-analysis of the effects of soy protein intake on serum lipids. N Engl J Med. 1995 Aug 3;333(5):276–282. [PubMed]

Bai W, Henneicke-von Zepelin HH, Wang S, Zheng S, Liu J, Zhang Z, et al. Efficacy and tolerability of a medicinal product containing an isopropanolic black cohosh extract in Chinese women with menopausal symptoms: a randomized, double blind, parallel-controlled study versus tibolone. *Maturitas.* 2007 Sep 20;58(1):31-41.

Bernardi M, D'Intino PE, Trevisani F, Cantelli-Forti G, Raggi MA, Turchetto E, Gasbarrini G. Effects of prolonged ingestion of graded doses of licorice by healthy volunteers. Life Sci.1994;55(11):863–872. [PubMed]

BLATT MHG, WIESBADER H, KUPPERMAN HS. Vitamin E and climacteric syndrome; failure of effective control as measured by menopausal index. AMA Arch Intern Med. 1953 Jun;91(6):792–799. [PubMed]

Briese V, Stammwitz U, Friede M, Henneicke-von Zepelin HH. Black cohosh with or without St. John's wort for symptom-specific climacteric treatment -- results of a large-scale, controlled, observational study. *Maturitas*. 2007 Aug 20;57(4):405-14.

Burr ML, Fehily AM, Gilbert JF, Rogers S, Holliday RM, Sweetnam PM, et al. Effects of changes in fat, fish, and fibre intakes on death and myocardial reinfarction. Lancet. 1989; 2:757–61.

Cahill DJ, Fox R, Wardle PG, Harlow CR. Multiple follicular development associated with herbal medicine. Hum Reprod. 1994 Aug;9(8):1469–1470. [PubMed]

Carroll DG. Nonhormonal Therapies for Hot Flashes in Menopause. American Family Physician: Vol. 73, No. 3: Feb 1, 2006, pp. 457-464.

Caso Marasco A, Vargas Ruiz R, Salas Villagomez A, Begoña Infante C. Double-blind study of a multivitamin complex supplemented with ginseng extract. Drugs Exp Clin Res. 1996;22(6):323–329. [PubMed]

Chandeying V, Sangthawan M. Efficacy comparison of Pueraria mirifica (PM) against conjugated equine estrogen (CEE) with/without medroxyprogesterone acetate (MPA) in the treatment of climacteric symptoms in perimenopausal women: phase III study. *J Med Assoc Thai*. 2007 Sep;90(9):1720-6.

Chenoy R, Hussain S, Tayob Y, O'Brien PM, Moss MY, Morse PF. Effect of oral gamolenic acid from evening primrose oil on menopausal flushing. BMJ. 1994 Feb 19;308(6927):501–503.[PMC free article] [PubMed]

Deshpande SS. Food legumes in human nutrition: a personal perspective. Crit Rev Food Sci Nutr.1992;32(4):333–363. [PubMed]

Dietary supplementation with n-3 polyunsaturated fatty acids and vitamin E after myocardial infarction: results of the GISSI-Prevenzione trial. Gruppo Italiano per lo Studio della Sopravvivenza nell'Infarto miocardico. Lancet 1999; 354:447–55.

Düker EM, Kopanski L, Jarry H, Wuttke W. Effects of extracts from Cimicifuga racemosa on gonadotropin release in menopausal women and ovariectomized rats. Planta Med. 1991 Oct;57(5):420–424. [PubMed]

Dwyer JT, Goldin BR, Saul N, Gualtieri L, Barakat S, Adlercreutz H. Tofu and soy drinks contain phytoestrogens. J Am Diet Assoc. 1994 Jul;94(7):739–743. [PubMed]

Einer-Jensen N, Zhao J, Andersen KP, Kristoffersen K. Cimicifuga and Melbrosia lack oestrogenic effects in mice and rats. Maturitas. 1996 Oct;25(2):149–153. [PubMed]

Gambacciani M, Spinetti A, Piaggesi L, Cappagli B, Taponeco F, Manetti P, Weiss C, Teti GC, La Commare P, Facchini V. Ipriflavone prevents the bone mass reduction in premenopausal women treated with gonadotropin hormone-releasing hormone agonists. Bone Miner. 1994 Jul;26(1):19–26. [PubMed]

Geller SE, Studee L. Soy and red clover for mid-life and aging. Climacteric 2006; 9:245-263.

Grady D et al. Cardiovascular disease outcomes during 6.8 years of hormone therapy: Heart and Estrogen/progestin Replacement Study follow-up (HERS II). JAMA July 3, 2002; 288(1):49-57.

Green J, Denham A, Ingram J, Hawkey S, Greenwood R. Treatment of menopausal symptoms by qualified herbal practitioners: a prospective, randomized controlled trial. *Fam Pract*. 2007 Oct;24(5):468-74.

Griffin R. Soy Instead of HRT? Maybe Not. Aug. 20, 2004. Available at: www.healthandage.com

Hertog MG, Kromhout D, Aravanis C, Blackburn H, Buzina R, Fidanza F, Giampaoli S, Jansen A, Menotti A, Nedeljkovic S, et al. Flavonoid intake and long-term risk of coronary heart disease and cancer in the seven countries study. Arch Intern Med. 1995 Feb 27;155(4):381–386. [PubMed]

Hidalgo LA, Chedraui PA, Morocho N, et al. The effect of red clover isoflavones on menopausal symptoms, lipids and vaginal cytology in menopausal women: A randomized, double-blind, placebo-controlled study. *Gynecol Endocrinol*. 2005;21:257-264.

Hirata JD, Swiersz LM, Zell B, Small R, Ettinger B. Does dong quai have estrogenic effects in postmenopausal women? A double-blind, placebo-controlled trial. Fertil Steril. 1997 Dec;68(6):981–986. [PubMed]

Hopkins MP, Androff L, Benninghoff AS. Ginseng face cream and unexplained vaginal bleeding.Am J Obstet Gynecol. 1988 Nov;159(5):1121–1122. [PubMed]

Horiuchi T et al. Effect of soy protein on bone metabolism in postmenopausal Japanese women. Osteoporosis International 2000; 11(8):721-4.

Huang MI, Nir Y, Chen B, et al. A randomized controlled pilot study of acupuncture for postmenopausal hot flashes: effect on nocturnal hot flashes and sleep quality. *Fertil Steril.* 2006;86:700-710.

Huxtable RJ, Awang DV. Pyrrolizidine poisoning. Am J Med. 1990 Oct;89(4):547–548.[PubMed]

Huxtable RJ. The myth of beneficent nature: the risks of herbal preparations. Ann Intern Med.1992 Jul 15;117(2):165–166. [PubMed]

Katan MB. Flavonoids and heart disease. Am J Clin Nutr. 1997 May;65(5):1542–1543. [PubMed]

Khoo SK, Munro C, Battistutta D. Evening primrose oil and treatment of premenstrual syndrome.Med J Aust. 1990 Aug 20;153(4):189–192. [PubMed]

Kleijnen J. Evening primrose oil. BMJ. 1994 Oct 1;309(6958):824–825. [PMC free article][PubMed]

Knight DC, Eden JA. A review of the clinical effects of phytoestrogens. Obstet Gynecol. 1996 May;87(5 Pt 2):897–904. [PubMed]

Knight DC, Eden JA. Phytoestrogens--a short review. Maturitas. 1995 Nov;22(3):167–175.[PubMed]

Kotsopoulos, D. et al. The effects of soy protein containing phytoestrogens on menopausal symptoms in postmenopausal women. Climacteric September 2000; 3(3):161-7.

Kreijkamp-Kaspers S, Kok L, Grobbee DE, et al. Effect of soy protein containing isoflavones on cognitive function, bone mineral density, and plasma lipids in postmenopausal women. *JAMA*. 2004;292:65-74.

Kronenberg F, Fugh-Berman. Complementary and alternative medicine for menopausal symptoms: A review of randomized, controlled trials. Annals of Internal Medicine November 19, 2002; 137(10):805-13.

Kurzer MS. Hormonal effects of soy isoflavones: studies in premenopausal and postmenopausal women. Journal of Nutrition March 2000; 130(3):660S-1S.

Lewis JE, et al. A randomized controlled trial of the effect of dietary soy and flaxseed muffins on quality of life and hot flashes during menopause. Menopause, Vol 13, No. 4 pp 631-642.

Lo AC, Chan K, Yeung JH, Woo KS. Danggui (Angelica sinensis) affects the pharmacodynamics but not the pharmacokinetics of warfarin in rabbits. Eur J Drug Metab Pharmacokinet. 1995 Jan-Mar;20(1):55–60. [PubMed]

Lock M. Contested meanings of the menopause. Lancet. 1991 May 25;337(8752):1270–1272.[PubMed]

Low Dog T. Menopause: a review of botanical dietary supplements. *The American Journal of Medicine*. 2005;118(12) Suppl 2.

Lucas M, Asselin G, Merette C, et al. Effects of ethyl-eicosapentaenoic acid omega-3 fatty acid supplementation on hot flashes and quality of life among middle-aged women: a double-blind, placebo-controlled, randomized clinical trial. *Menopause*. 2009;16:357-66.

Lund K. Menopause and the Menopausal Transition. *Medical Clinics of North America*. 2008;92(5).

Ma J et al. U.S. women desire greater professional guidance on hormone and alternative therapies for menopause symptom management. Menopause: Vol 13, No. 3, pp 506-516.

McLAREN HC. Vitamin E in the menopause. Br Med J. 1949 Dec 17;2(4641):1378–illust.[PMC free article] [PubMed]

Miksicek RJ. Commonly occurring plant flavonoids have estrogenic activity. Mol Pharmacol. 1993 Jul;44(1):37–43. [PubMed]

Milewicz A, Gejdel E, Sworen H, Sienkiewicz K, Jedrzejak J, Teucher T, Schmitz H. Vitex agnus castus-Extrakt zur Behandlung von Regeltempoanomalien infolge latenter Hyperprolaktinämie. Ergebnisse einer randomisierten Plazebo-kontrollierten Doppelblindstudie.Arzneimittelforschung. 1993 Jul;43(7):752–756. [PubMed]

Morrelli V, Naquin C. Alternative Therapies for Tradiational Disease States: Menopause. American Family Physician 2002: 66. Available at: www.aafp.org

Murkies AL, Lombard C, Strauss BJ, Wilcox G, Burger HG, Morton MS. Dietary flour supplementation decreases post-menopausal hot flushes: effect of soy and wheat. Maturitas. 1995 Apr;21(3):189–195. [PubMed]

Nagata C et al. Soy protein intake and hot flashes in Japanese women: results from a community-based prospective study. American Journal of Epidemiology April 15, 2000; 153(8):790-3.

Natural Medicines: Comprehensive Database. Therapeutic Research Faculty, 2002.

Nelson HD et al. Nonhormonal Therapies for Menopausal Hot Flashes: a systematic review and meta-analysis. JAMA May 3, 2006: Vol 295, No 17, pp 2057-71.

Nelson HD et al. Postmenopausal hormone replacement therapy: a scientific review. JAMA August 21, 2002; 288(7):872-81.

Nestel PJ, Pomeroy S, Kay S, Komesaroff P, Behrsing J, Cameron JD, et al. Isoflavones from red clover improve systemic arterial compliance but not plasma lipids in menopausal women. J Clin Endocrinol Metab. 1999;84:895–8.

O'Keefe JH, Harris WS. From inuit to implementation: omega-3 fatty acids come of age. Mayo Clin Proc. 2000;75:607–14.

Osmers R, Friede M, Liske E, et al. Efficacy and safety of isopropanolic black cohosh extract for climacteric symptoms. *Obstet Gynecol.* 2005;105:1074-1083.

Ozaki Y, Ma JP. Inhibitory effects of tetramethylpyrazine and ferulic acid on spontaneous movement of rat uterus in situ. Chem Pharm Bull (Tokyo) 1990 Jun;38(6):1620–1623. [PubMed]

Pockaj BA, Gallagher JG, Loprinzi CL, et al. Phase III Double-Blind, Randomized, Placebo-Controlled Crossover Trial of Black Cohosh in the Management of Hot Flashes: NCCTG Trial N01CC1. *J Clin Oncol.* 2006;24:2836-2841.

Potter SM, Baum JA, Tong H, Stillman RJ, Shay NF, Erdmfan JW Jr. Soy protein and isoflavones: their effects on blood lipids and bone density in postmenopausal women. Am J Clin Nutr. 1998;68(6 Suppl):1375S–9S.

Poulsen RC, Moughan PJ, Kruger MC. Long-chain polyunsaturated fatty acids and the regulation of bone metabolism. *Exp Biol Med* (Maywood). 2007 Nov;232(10):1275-88. Review.

Pruthi S, Thompson SL, Novotny PJ, Barton DL, Kottschade LA, Tan AD, et al. Pilot evaluation of flaxseed for the management of hot flashes. *J Soc Integr Oncol.* 2007 Summer;5(3):106-12.

Punnonen R, Lukola A. Oestrogen-like effect of ginseng. Br Med J. 1980 Oct 25;281(6248):1110–1110. [PMC free article] [PubMed]

Pye JK, Mansel RE, Hughes LE. Clinical experience of drug treatments for mastalgia. Lancet.1985 Aug 17;2(8451):373–377. [PubMed]

Rani S. The psychosexual implications of menopause. *Br J Nurs.* 2009;18(6):370-3.

Reid IR, Ames RW, Evans MC, Gamble GD, Sharpe SJ. Effect of calcium supplementation on bone loss in postmenopausal women. N Engl J Med. 1993 Feb 18;328(7):460–464. [PubMed]

Robien K, Cutler GJ, Lazovich D. Vitamin D intake and breast cancer risk in postmenopausal women: the Iowa Women's Health Study. *Cancer Causes Control.* 2007 Sep;18(7):775-82.

Rude RK, Kirchen ME, Gruber HE, Stasky RA, Meyer MH. Magnesium deficiency induces bone loss in the rat. Miner Electrolyte Metab. 1998;24:314–20.

Sacks FM et al. Soy Protein, Isoflavones, and Cardiovascular Health: An American Heart Association Science Advisory for Professionals From the Nutrition Committee. Circulation. 2006; 113:1034-1044.

Scheiber MD, Rebar RW. Isoflavones and postmenopausal bone health: a viable alternative to estrogen therapy?. Menopause. 1999;6:233–41.

Schubert W, Cullberg G, Edgar B, Hedner T. Inhibition of 17 beta-estradiol metabolism by grapefruit juice in ovariectomized women. Maturitas. 1994 Dec;20(2-3):155–163. [PubMed]

Secreto G, Chiechi LM, Amadori A, et al. Soy isoflavones and melatonin for the relief of climacteric symptoms: a multicenter, double-blind, randomized study. *Maturitas.* 2004;47:11-20.

Seibel M. The Soy Solution for Menopause – The Estrogen Alternative. 2003. Simon & Schuster: NYNY.

Singh RB, Niaz MA, Sharma JP, Kumar R, Rastpgo V, Moshirl M. Randomized, double-blind, placebo-controlled trial of fish oil and mustard oil in patients with suspected acute myocardial infarction: the Indian experiment of infarct survival—4. Cardiovasc Drugs Ther. 1997; 11:485–91.

Sliutz G, Speiser P, Schultz AM, Spona J, Zeillinger R. Agnus castus extracts inhibit prolactin secretion of rat pituitary cells. Horm Metab Res. 1993 May;25(5):253–255. [PubMed]

Somjen D, Knoll E, Vaya J, et al. Estrogen-like activity of licorice root constituents: glabridin and glabrene, in vascular tissues in vitro and in vivo. *J Steroid Biochem Mol Biol.* 2004;91:147-155.

Spangler L, Newton KM, Grothaus LC, Reed SD, Ehrlich K, LaCroix AZ. The effects of black cohosh therapies on lipids, fibrinogen, glucose and insulin. *Maturitas.* 2007 Jun 20;57(2):195-204.

St. Germaine A et al. Isoflavone-rich or isoflavone-poor soy protein does not reduce menopausal symptoms during 24 weeks of treatment. Menopause January-February 2001; 8(1):17-26.

Tamaya T, Sato S, Okada H. Inhibition by plant herb extracts of steroid bindings in uterus, liver and serum of the rabbit. Acta Obstet Gynecol Scand. 1986;65(8):839–842. [PubMed]

Trock BJ et al. Meta-Analysis of Soy Intake and Breast Cancer Risk. Journal of the National Cancer Institute, Vol. 98, No. 7, pp 459-471.

Tucker KL, Hannan MT, Chen H, Cupples LA, Wilson PW, Kiel DP. Potassium, magnesium, and fruit and vegetable intakes are associated with greater bone mineral density in elderly men and women. Am J Clin Nutr. 1999;69:727–36.

Uebelhack R, Blohmer JU, Graubaum HJ, et al. Black cohosh and St. John's wort for climacteric complaints: a randomized trial.*Obstet Gynecol.* 2006;107:247-255.

Unfer V et al. Endometrial effects of long-term treatment with phytoestrogens: a randomized, double-blind, placebo-controlled study. Fertility and Sterility: Vol. 82, Issue 1, July 2004, pp 145-148.

Valente M, Bufalino L, Castiglione GN, D'Angelo R, Mancuso A, Galoppi P, Zichella L. Effects of 1-year treatment with ipriflavone on bone in postmenopausal women with low bone mass. Calcif Tissue Int. 1994 May;54(5):377–380. [PubMed]

Viana M, Barbas C, Bonet B, Bonet MV, Castro M, Fraile MV, Herrera E. In vitro effects of a flavonoid-rich extract on LDL oxidation. Atherosclerosis. 1996 Jun;123(1-2):83–91. [PubMed]

Vigna GB et al. Plasma lipoproteins in soy-treated postmenopausal women: a double-blind, placebo-controlled trial. Nutr Metab Cardiovasc Dis December 2000; 10(6):315-22.

Vincent A, Fitzpatrick LA. Soy isoflavones: are they useful in menopause? Mayo Clin Proc November 2000; 75(11):1174-84. www.mayoclinic.com

Wilcox G, Wahlqvist ML, Burger HG, Medley G. Oestrogenic effects of plant foods in postmenopausal women. BMJ. 1990 Oct 20;301(6757):905–906. [PMC free article] [PubMed]

Wuttke W, Jarry H, Seidlová-Wuttke D. Isoflavones -- safe food additives or dangerous drugs? *Ageing Res Rev.* 2007 Aug;6(2):150-88.

Yang HM, Liao MF, Zhu SY, et al. A randomised, double-blind, placebo-controlled trial on the effect of Pycnogenol on the climacteric syndrome in peri-menopausal women. *Acta Obstet Gynecol Scand.* 2007;86:978-85.

Zaborowska E, Brynhildsen J, Damberg S, et al. Effects of acupuncture, applied relaxation, estrogens, and placebo on hot flushes in postmenopausal women: an analysis of two prospective, parallel, randomized studies. *Climacteric.* 2007;10:38-45.

Articles

Ant, M. Diabetic vulvovaginitis treated with vitamin E suppositories. American Journal of Obstetrics and Gynecology 1954; 67:407.

Band, P. R., et al. Treatment of benign breast disease with vitamin A. Preventive Medicine 1984; 13:549.

Biskind, M. S., and G. R. Biskind. Effect of vitamin B complex deficiency on inactivation of estrone in the liver. Endocrinology 1942; 31:109.

Biskind, M. S. Nutritional deficiency in the etiology of menorrhagia, cystic mastitis and premenstrual tension, treatment with vitamin B complex. Journal of Clinical Endocrinology and Metabolism 1943; 3:227.

Block, G. Vitamin C and cancer prevention. The epidemiologic evidence. American Journal of Clinical Nutrition 1991; 53:2701.

Brattstrom, L. E., et al. Folic acid responsive postmenopausal homocysteinemia. Metabolism 1985; 34:1073.

Breast Cancer Prevention Group. Breast cancer environmental factors. The Lancet 1992; 340:904.

Bullock, C., Soybeans: an ERT alternative. Medical Tribune 1995; p. 11.

Cheng, E. W., et al. Estrogenic activity of some naturally occurring isoflavones. Annals of New York Academy of Sciences 1955; 61(3):652.

Christy, C. J. Vitamin E in menopause. Preliminary report of experimental and clinical study. American Journal of Obstetrics and Gynecology 1945; 50:84.

Clemetson, C. A. B., et al. Capillary strength and the menstrual cycle. New York Academy of Sciences 1962; 93(7):277.

Cohen, J. D., and H. W. Rubin. Functional menorrhagia. Treatment with bioflavonoids and vitamin C. Current Therapeutic Research 1960; 2(11):539.

Cordova, C., et al. Influence of ascorbic acid on platelet aggregation in vitro and in vivo. Atherosclerosis 1981; 41:15.

Dawson-Hughes, B., et al. A controlled trial of the effect of calcium supplementation on bone density in postmenopausal women. New England Journal of Medicine 1990; 323 (13):878.

Eskin, E. A., et al. Mammary gland dysplasia and iodine deficiency. Journal of the American Medical Association 1967; 200:115.

Finkler, R. S. The effect of vitamin E in the menopause. Journal of Clinical Endocrinology 1949; 9:89.

Gerster, K. Potential role of beta carotene in the prevention of cardiovascular disease. International Journal of Vitamin and Nutrities Research 1991; 61:277-91.

Goldin, B. R., et al. Effect of diet on excretion of estrogens in pre- and postmenopausal women. Cancer Research 1981; 41:3771.

Goldin, B. R., et al. Estrogen excretion patterns and plasma levels in vegetarian and omnivorous women. New England Journal of Medicine 1982; 307:1542.

Goodnight, S. H. The effects of Omega-3 fatty acids on thrombosis and atherogenesis. Hematologic Pathology 1989; 3(1):1.

Goodnight, S. H. Assessment of the therapeutic use of N-3 fatty acids in vascular disease and thrombosis Chest. 1991; 102(4):3745.

Gozan, H. A. The use of vitamin E in the treatment of menopause. New York State Medical Journal 1952; 15:1289.

Hain, A. M., and J. C. B. Sym. The control of menopausal flushes by vitamin E. British Medicine Journal 1943; 7:9.

Hasling, C., et al. Calcium metabolism in post menopausal osteoporotic women is determined by dietary calcium and coffee intake. Journal of Nutrition 1991; 112:1119- 1126.

Heaney, R. P. et al. Effect of calcium on skeletal development, bone loss and wrist fractures. The American Journal of Medicine 1991; 5B-23S-5B-28S.

Hennekens, C. A., et al. Beta carotene and cardiovascular disease. Beyond deficiency. New views on the functions and health effects of vitamins. New York Academy of Sciences. 1992; 22.

Henson, D. L., et al. Ascorbic acid. Biological functions and relation to cancer. Journal of The National Cancer Institute 1991; 83(8):547-50.

Horrobin, D. F Essential fatty acids and the complications of diabetes mellitus. Wien Klin Wochenschr 1989; 101(8):289.

Horrobin, D. F. Essential fatty acids in clinical dermatology. Journal of the American Academy of Dermatology 1987 20(6):1045.

Horrobin, D. E The regulation of prostaglandin biosynthesis by the manipulation of essential fatty acid metabolism. Revue of Pure and Applied Pharmacologic Science 1980; 4(4):339.

Howe, G. R., et al. Dietary factors and the risk of breast cancer. Combined analysis of 12 case-controlled studies. Journal of The National Cancer Institute 1990; 82:561-9.

Hunter, D. T. Antioxidant micronutrients and breast cancer. Journal of the American College of Nutrition 1992; 11(5):633.

Kavinovsky, N. R. Vitamin E and the control of climacteric symptoms. Annals of Western Medicine and Surgery 1950; 4(1):27.

Kellis, T., and L. E. Vickery. Inhibition of human estrogen synthetase (aromatase) by flavones. Science 1984; 225:1032-4.

Licato, A. Effect of supplemental calcium on serum and urinary calcium in osteoporotic patients. Journal of the American College of Nutrition 1992; 11(2):164-7.

Lithgow, P. M., and W. M. Politzer. Vitamin A in the treatment of menorrhagia. South African Medical Journal 1977; 51:191.

London, R. S., et al. Endocrine parameters in alpha-tocopheryl therapy of patients with mammary dysplasia. Cancer Research 1981; 41:3811.

London, R. S., et al. Mammary dysplasia. Clinical response and urinary excretion of 11-deoxy-17-ketosteroids and pregnanediol following alpha-tocopherol therapy. Breast 1976; 4:19.

Lutz, J. Calcium balance and acid base status of women as affected by increased protein intake and by sodium bicarbonate ingestion. American Journal of Clinical Nutrition 1984; 39:20.

Manson, T., et al. A prospective study of vitamin C and the incidence of coronary heart disease in women. Circulation 1992; 85:865.

McKeown, L. A. Diet high in fruits and vegetables linked to lower breast cancer risk. Medical Tribune 1992; 9:14.

McLaren, H. C. Vitamin E in the menopause. British Medical Journal 1949; 12:1378.

Osilesi, 0., et al. Blood pressure and plasma lipids during ascorbic acid supplementation to borderline hypertensive and normotensive adults. Nutrition Research 1991; 11:405-12.

Pauling, L. Prevention and treatment of heart disease. New research focus at the Linus Pauling Institute. Linus Pauling Institute of Science and Medicine Newsletter 1992; 1.

Pauling, L. How vitamin C can prevent heart attack and stroke. Linus Pauling Institute for Science and Medicine Newsletter 1992; 3.

Pauling, L. Vitamin C and heart disease. A chronology. Linus Pauling Institute for Science and Medicine Newsletter 1992; 2.

Pope, G. S., et al. Isolation of oestrogenic isoflavone (biochanin A) from red clover. Chemistry and Industry 1953; 10:1042.

Potischman, N. Association between breast cancer, plasma triglycerides and cholesterol. Nutrition and Cancer 1991; 15:205-15.

Preuter, G. W. A treatment for excessive uterine bleeding. Applied Therapeutics 1961; 5:351.

Shute, E. V., et al. The influence of vitamin E on vascular disease. Surgery, Gynecology and Obstetrics 1948; 86:1.

Simard, A. Nutrition and lifestyle factors in fibrocystic disease and cancer of the breast. Cancer Prevention and Nutrition 1990; 567-72.

Simin, T. Vitamin C and cardiovascular disease. A review. The American College of Nutrition 1992; 11(2):107-25.

Singer, E. Effects of vitamin E deficiency on the thyroid gland of the rat. Journal of Physiology 1936; 87:287.

Smith, C. J. Nonhormonal control of vaso-motor flushing in menopausal patients. Chicago Medicine 1964; 67:193.

Solomon, D., et al. Relationship between vitamin E and urinary excretion of ketosteroid fractions in cystic mastitis. Annals of New York Academy of Sciences 1972; 2(3):103.

Taylor, F A. Habitual abortion. Therapeutic evaluation of citrus bioflavonoids. Western Journal of Surgery, Obstetrics and Gynecology 1956; 5:286.

Van Beresteijn, E. Habitual dietary calcium intake and cortical bone loss in perimenopausal women. A longitudinal study. Calcified Tissue International 1990; 47:338-44.

Watson, E. M. Clinical experiences with wheat germ oil (vitamin E). Canadian Medical Association Journal 1936; 2:134.

Weaver, C. M. Calcium bioavailability and its relationship to osteoporosis. Proceedings for the Society of Experimental Biology and Medicine 1992; 200:157-60.

Wertz, P W., et al. Essential fatty acids and epidermal integrity. Archives of Dermatology 1987; 123(10):1381.

Whitacre, F E., and B. Barrera. War amenorrhea. Journal of the American Medical Association 1944; 124:399.

Wilcox, G., et al. Estrogen effects of plant foods in postmenopausal women. British Medical Journal 1990; 301:905-6.

Zardize, D. G. Fatty acid composition of phospholipids in erythrocyte membranes and risk of breast cancer. International Journal of Cancer 1990; 45:807-10.

Ziegler, T., Soybeans show promise in cancer prevention. News from the National Cancer Institute 1995; p.11-12.

Baranov, A. I. Medicinal uses of ginseng and related plants in the Soviet Union: Recent trends in the Soviet literature. Journal of Ethnopharmacology 1982; 6:339-53.

Costello, C. H., and E. V. Lynn. Estrogenic substances from plants. I. Glycyrrhiza. Journal of the American Pharmaceutical Society 1950. 39:177-80.

Chen, E. W., et al. Estrogenic activity of some naturally occurring isoflavones. Annals of the New York Academy of Sciences 1955. 61(3):652

Cohen, J. D., and H. W. Rubin. Functional menorrhagia: Treatment with bioflavonoids and vitamin C. Current Therapeutic Research 1960. 2(11):539.

Dansi, A., et al. The estrogenic activity of polymerized anol. Biochimica e Terapia Sperimentale 1937. 24:282-4.

Dodds, E. C., and W. Lawson. Estrogenic activity of p-hydroxypropenyl-benzene (anol). Nature 1937. 139:1039.

Dodds, E. C., and W. Lawson. A simple oestrogenic agent with an activity of the same order as that of oestrone. Nature 1937. 139:627.

Elghamry, M. I., and I. M. Shihata. Biological activity of phytoestrogens. Planta Medica 1965. 13:352-7.

Gibson, M. R. Glycyrrhiza in old and new perspectives. Lloydia 1978. 41:348-54.

Gomez, E. T., and C. W. Turner. Effect of anol and dihydrotheelin on mammogenic activity of the pituitary gland of rabbits. Proceedings of the Society for Experimental Biology and Medicine 1938. 39:140-42.

Kuhnau, J. The flavonoids: A class of semi-essential food components: Their role in human nutrition. World Review of Nutrition and Diet 1976. 24:117-91.

Leathwood, P. D., and F Chauffard. Aqueous extract of valerian reduces latency to fall asleep in man. Planta Medica 1985. 54:144-8.

Leathwood, P. D., et al. Aqueous extract of valerian root (Valeriani Officinalis L.) improves sleep quality in man. Pharmacol. Biochem Behavior 1982. 17:65-71.

Pearse, H. A., and J. D. Trisler. A rational approach to the treatment of habitual abortion and menometorrhagia. Clinical Medicine 1957. 9:1081.

Pope, G. S., et al. Isolation of an oestrogenic isoflavone (Biochanin A) from red clover. Chemistry and Industry 1953. 10:1042.

Preuter, G. W. A treatment for excessive uterine bleeding. Applied Therapeutics 1961. 5:351.

Schumann, E. Newer concepts of blood coagulation and control of hemorrhage. American Journal of Obstetrics and Gynecology 1939. 38:1002-7.

Suekawa, M., et al. Pharmacological studies on ginger. I. pharmacological actions of pungent constituents, (6) gingerol and (6) shogaol. Journal of Pharmacologic Dynamics 1984. 7:836-48.